Surgical Techniques in Sports Medicine

Foot and Ankle Surgery

Surgical Techniques in Sports Medicine

Foot and Ankle Surgery

Gian Luigi Canata MD
Director and Orthopaedic Surgeon
Centre for Sports Traumatology and Arthroscopic Surgery
Koelliker Hospital
Turin, Italy

Lee Parker BM, MRCS (Eng), FRCS(Tr&Orth)
Consultant Trauma and Orthopaedic Foot and Ankle Surgeon
The Royal London Hospital
London, UK

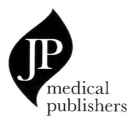

JP
medical
publishers

London • Philadelphia • Panama City • New Delhi

© 2016 JP Medical Ltd.
Published by JP Medical Ltd
83 Victoria Street, London, SW1H 0HW, UK
Tel: +44 (0)20 3170 8910
Fax: +44 (0)20 3008 6180
Email: info@jpmedpub.com
Web: www.jpmedpub.com

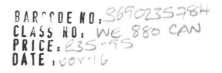

The rights of Gian Luigi Canata and Lee Parker to be identified as editors of this work have been asserted by them in accordance with the Copyright, Designs and Patents Act 1988.

ISBN: 978-1-909836-34-1

British Library Cataloguing in Publication Data
A catalogue record for this book is available from the British Library

Library of Congress Cataloging in Publication Data
A catalog record for this book is available from the Library of Congress

Commissioning Editor: Steffan Clements
Development Editor: Gavin Smith
Design: Designers Collective Ltd

Foreword

Education is one of the key missions of EFOST, the European Federation of National Associations of Orthopaedic Sports Traumatology. The *Surgical Techniques in Sports Medicine* series is the educational flagship of EFOST, and provides an invaluable supplement to the experience afforded by the international EFOST Travelling Fellowship.

This series of highly illustrated handbooks, each dedicated to a specific anatomical region, is aimed at established surgeons, fellows in orthopaedic sports traumatology and residents in orthopaedics. It comprises much more than the simple scientific evidence behind each procedure. The aim instead is to impart practical knowledge arising from the direct experience of highly skilled surgeons, who describe reliable surgical procedures in a practical, easy-to-follow manner that will be of great value to orthopaedic and sports trauma surgeons alike.

Surgical Techniques in Sports Medicine is the fruit of five years' work by the three immediate past presidents of EFOST and is testament to how far EFOST has come since its foundation in 1992.

We hope that you find this book, and the others in the series, a useful resource.

Gernot Felmet
President, EFOST
Nicola Maffulli
Series Editor
François Kelberine
Series Editor

October 2015

Contents

Contributors

Enrico Balboni, MD
Orthopaedic Surgeon
Centre for Sports Traumatology
Ospedale Koelliker
Turin, Italy

Ignazio Bagnoli, MD
Clinica Cellini
Turin, Italy

Donato M Bardelli, MD
Orthopaedic Surgeon
Centre for Sports Traumatology
Ospedale Koelliker
Turin, Italy

Marco Bargagliotti, MD
Department of Sports and Orthopaedic Surgery
IRCCS Policlinico San Matteo
University of Pavia
Pavia, Italy

Francesco Benazzo, MD
Professor of Orthopaedics and Traumatology
Surgery
Department of Sports and Orthopaedic Surgery
IRCCS Policlinico San Matteo
University of Pavia
Pavia, Italy

Roberto Buda, MD
Professor of Orthopaedic Surgery
Orthopaedic and Traumatology Clinic I
Rizzoli Orthopaedic Institute
Bologna, Italy

Gian Luigi Canata, MD
Director, Centre for Sports Traumatology
Koelliker Hospital
Turin, Italy

Silvio Caravelli, MD
Orthopaedic Surgeon
Orthopaedic and Traumatology Clinic I
Rizzoli Orthopaedic Institute
Bologna, Italy

Luca Carboni, MD
Orthopaedic Surgeon
Orthopaedic and Traumatology Clinic I
Rizzoli Orthopaedic Institute
Bologna, Italy

Valentina Casale, MD
Medical Doctor
Centre for Sports Traumatology
Koelliker Hospital
Turin, Italy

Francesco Castagnini, MD
Orthopaedic Surgeon
Orthopaedic and Traumatology Clinic I
Rizzoli Orthopaedic Institute
Bologna, Italy

Raul Cerlon, MD
Orthopaedic Surgeon
Orthopaedic Clinic I
University of Turin
Turin, Italy

Daniel V Comba, MD
Consultant Orthopaedic Surgeon
Orthopaedic Surgery Unit A
Koelliker Hospital
Sports Medicine Department
Clinica Fornaca
Turin, Italy

Alberto Combi, MD
Department of Sports and Orthopaedic Surgery
IRCCS Policlinico San Matteo
University of Pavia
Pavia, Italy

Giuseppe G Costa, MD
Orthopaedic Surgeon
Orthopaedic and Traumatology Clinic I
Rizzoli Orthopaedic Institute
Bologna, Italy

Walter Daghino, MD
Clinica Ortopedica dell'Università di Torino
Città della Salute e della Scienza
Turin, Italy

Angelo De Carli, MD
Professor of Orthopaedic Surgery
Department of Orthopaedic Surgery
Sant'Andrea Hospital
University of Rome
Rome, Italy

Iftach Hetsroni, MD
Orthopaedic Surgeon
Department of Orthopaedics – Meir Medical Center
Affiliated to Sacker School of Medicine, Tel Aviv
University
Kfar Saba, Israel

Andrew Hughes BM FRCS(Tr&Orth) FEBOT MSc
The Alfred Hospital
Melbourne, Australia

Lucky Jeyaseelan MBBS BSc MRCS
Specialist Trainee in Trauma and Orthopaedic
Surgery
The Royal London Hospital
London, UK

Charlie Jowett FRCS(Orth)
Foot and Ankle Fellow
The Alfred Hospital
Melbourne, Australia

Andrea Losana, MD
Orthopaedic Surgeon
Centre for Sports Traumatology
Ospedale Koelliker
Turin, Italy

Gideon Mann, MD
Orthopaedic Surgeon
Department of Orthopaedics – Meir Medical Center
Affiliated to Sacker School of Medicine, Tel Aviv
University
Kfar Saba, Israel

Marco Marcarelli, MD
Orthopaedic Surgeon
Ospedale Santa Croce
Moncalieri, Italy

Massimo Marconetto, MD
Orthopedic Surgeon, Foot and Ankle Surgery
Ospedale Santa Croce
Moncalieri, Italy

Simone Massimi, MD
Orthopaedic Surgeon
Orthopaedics and Traumatology Clinic I
Rizzoli Orthopaedic Institute
Bologna, Italy

Marco Messina, MD
Orthopaedic Specialist
Orthopaedic Clinic I, University of Turin
Turin, Italy
Orthopaedic Clinic, Hospital Vittorio Emanuele
Catania, Italy

Luigi Milano, MD
Clinica Cellini
Turin, Italy

Federico Morelli, MD
Professor of Orthopaedic Surgery
Orthopaedic Surgery
Sant'Andrea Hospital
University of Rome
Rome, Italy

Meir Nyska, MD
Orthopaedic Surgeon
Department of Orthopaedic Surgery – Meir Medical
Center
Affiliated to Sacker School of Medicine, Tel Aviv
University
Kfar Saba, Israel

Ezequiel Palmanovich, MD
Orthopaedic Surgeon
Department of Orthopaedic Surgery – Meir Medical
Center
Affiliated to Sacker School of Medicine, Tel Aviv
University
Kfar Saba, Israel

Enrico Parino, MD
Orthopaedic Surgeon
Orthopaedic Department
Maria Pia Hospital
Turin, Italy

Claudia Pesce, MD
Orthopaedic Surgeon
Centre for Sports Traumatology
Ospedale Koelliker
Turin, Italy

Sarah Rubin MBBSS MRCS
Specialist Trainee in Trauma and Orthopaedic
Surgery
Newham University Hospital
London, UK

Zacharia Silk BSc MBBS MRCS
Specialist Trainee in Trauma and Orthopaedic
Surgery,
Percivall Pott Rotation
Princess Alexandra Hospital
Harlow, UK

Kalpesh R Vaghela MBBS BSc MRCS PgCertME
Specialist Trainee in Trauma and Orthopaedic
Surgery
Percivall Pott Rotation
North East Thames
London, UK

Angiola Valente, MD
Clinica Cellini
Turin, Italy

Francesca Vannini, MD, PhD
Rizzoli Orthopaedic Institute
Bologna University
Bologna, Italy

Giacomo Zanon, MD
Department of Sports and Orthopaedic Surgery
IRCCS Policlinico San Matteo
University of Pavia
Pavia, Italy

Modified Broström procedure for lateral ligament repair

Indications

- Symptomatic, recurrent lateral ankle ligament sprains
- Failure of ankle instability to resolve despite physiotherapy to restore peroneal strength and ankle proprioception

Contraindications

- Fixed coronal hindfoot malalignment
- Degenerative and inflammatory joint disease
- Neuromuscular disorders (hereditary motor sensory neuropathy, peroneal nerve palsy)
- High body mass index
- Rear foot varus

Preoperative assessment

Clinical assessment

- Patients describe the perception of an unstable ankle
- Pain and swelling are often localized to the lateral side of the ankle (**Figure 1.1**)
- There is avoidance of aggravating activities such as walking on uneven surfaces or certain sports
- There may be coexistent peroneal tendinopathy related to an overuse phenomenon or a talar dome osteochondral lesion, giving rise to a deep-seated pain within the ankle
- Altered sensation or sensitivity may occur in the anterolateral foot due to stretching of the superficial peroneal nerve after recurrent sprains

Physical examination

- A comparative assessment of both ankles should be performed
- Lower limb and hindfoot alignment must be evaluated with the patient standing
- Gait should be assessed for obvious instability or antalgia
- A heel raise test should be performed, looking for normal hindfoot motion from valgus to varus, which is absent in patients with tarsal coalition
- Stability and proprioceptive control of the ankle may be evaluated with the patient undertaking a single-leg stance (Guillo, 2013)
- Tenderness to palpation is commonly detected beneath the fibular tip and on the anterolateral aspect of the ankle
- Joint motion should always be compared to the opposite side. Combined motion of the ankle and subtalar joints is evaluated by assessing the angle between the hindfoot and leg while inversion stress is applied to the calcaneum
- Isolation of subtalar motion requires the ankle to be held in dorsiflexion, thereby wedging the talus in the ankle mortise. Upon hindfoot inversion the calcaneus shifts medially to the talus if there is significant subtalar instability (Colville, 1998)
- Anterior drawer and talar tilt tests are performed and compared with the opposite limb for the assessment of ankle stability
- Talar tilt test: the angle formed by tibial plafond and talar dome is measured applying an inversion force to the talus while stabilizing the distal part of leg with the other hand

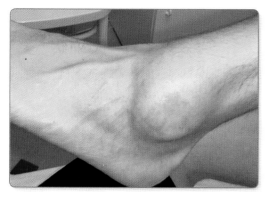

Figure 1.1 Symptomatic ankle: pain and swelling.

- Assess generalized joint laxity using the Beighton Score
- The clinician should also test the strength and integrity of the peroneal tendons
- A neurovascular assessment of the foot is also recommended

Imaging assessment

Radiographs

- Standard plain radiographs include standing anteroposterior, lateral, and mortise views, and a Saltzman or Meary view
- Comparative stress radiographs with anterior drawer and varus tilt may be performed. Radiographs are useful to help identify contributory pathology such as bone spurs and osteochondral lesions of the talus (Colville, 1998)

Magnetic resonance imaging (MRI)

- When deep pain occurs suggesting an oseochondral lesion, MRI is useful to assess the grade and severity
- MRI may also highlight the torn or stretched lateral ligament complex

Ultrasonography

- Ultrasonography may be useful in the investigation of tendon pathology

Computed tomography (CT)

- CT or MRI-arthrography is not usually performed, but can be helpful for detailed assessment of cystic osteochondral lesions

Timing for surgery

- Surgery takes place when swelling permits
- Muscles and tendons of the leg should ensure adequate stability, excluding the ligamentous injury
- There should be a normal range of ankle motion

Surgical preparation

Special surgical considerations

- It is useful to perform ankle arthroscopy before repair of the lateral ligament complex. Up to 95% of patients undergoing surgery for lateral ankle instability have associated intra-articular pathology (Ferkel, 2007)
- Consider performing a simultaneous lateralizing calcaneal osteotomy for patients with hindfoot varus deformity

Surgical equipment

Arthroscopic equipment

- Arthroscope: 2.7 mm or 4.5 mm 30°-angled
- Light source and cables
- Camera system and monitor
- Arthroscopic probe (hook)
- Arthroscopic punches (basket forceps)
- Arthroscopic grasper
- Motorized shaver
- Noninvasive ankle distractor
- Gravity system or pump for instillation of 0.9% saline
- Microfracture picks

Open surgery equipment

- Needle holder
- Sutures
- Scalpel, blades no. 11 and 21
- Forceps: toothed tissue forceps, Adson's tissue forceps, Kocher's, Kelly's and mosquito forceps
- Scissors
- Luer bone rongeur
- Farabeuf retractors
- Mini Hohmann bone elevators
- Bone curettes
- Hand drill
- Drill guide
- Kirschner (K)-wires

Equipment positioning

- The arthroscopic tower is positioned on the opposite side of the ankle, at the level of patient's contralateral hip
- The open surgery equipment is positioned near the surgeon, at the same side of the ankle that is being operated

Patient positioning

- Position the patient supine with the knee extended
- A well-padded tourniquet is placed on the proximal lower thigh; some surgeons may choose not to inflate the tourniquet during arthroscopy
- A sandbag under the ipsilateral buttock allows improved access to both the lateral and medial sides of the ankle. The heel should be on the end of the operating table
- Initially, no ankle distraction is applied and an examination under anesthetic is performed to assess stability

Further preparation

- The patient receives a single dose of intravenous antibiotics preoperatively
- The procedure is preferably performed under general anesthesia but can be performed with a regional nerve block

Surgical technique

Ankle arthroscopy

- It is important to treat any concomitant pathology such as osteochondral lesions (**Figure 1.2**)
- An anteromedial portal is established medial to the tibialis anterior tendon at the level of the tibiotalar joint using a 'nick and spread' technique
- With the arthroscope in the standard anteromedial portal, the superficial peroneal nerve can be identified by directing the light source externally. The anterolateral portal is then established lateral to the peroneus tertius tendon
- Noninvasive ankle distraction can be applied to the ankle to improve access, and with these portals the majority of talar dome osteochondral lesions, distal tibial bone spurs, and soft tissue impingements can be addressed

Open procedure

Tissue dissection

- The arthroscope and any distraction should be removed from the ankle before the ligament repair commences
- The surgical incision passes longitudinally for 3 cm over the distal fibula and proceeds in a J-shape with the incision turning 45° toward the talar neck. Care should be exercised to avoid cutting the peroneal tendons
- Along the course of the incision there are branches of the short saphenous vein which require cautery with diathermy or ligation. It is important to avoid the lateral cutaneous branch of the superficial peroneal nerve passing anterior to the distal fibula
- The peroneal tendons can be explored by extending this surgical approach. Otherwise they are retracted posteriorly, exposing the capsule (**Figures 1.3** and **1.4**)
- The capsule–ligamentous complex along the anterior distal fibula is incised, leaving a 3–5 mm cuff on the outermost aspect of the fibula

Ligament plication

- The anterior talofibular ligament (ATFL) is identified as a slight thickening in the capsule passing horizontally toward the talar neck.

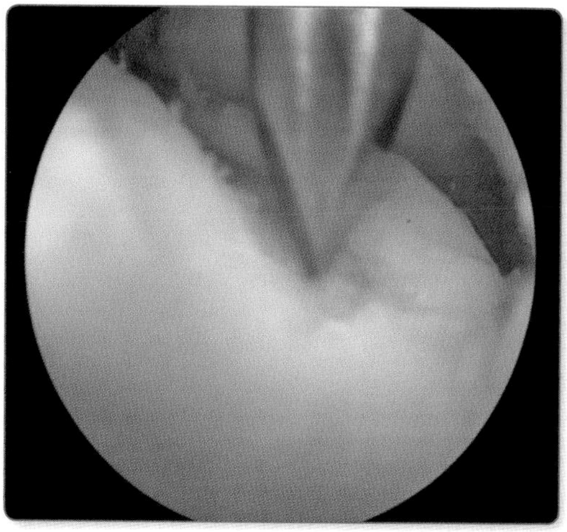

Figure 1.2 Microfracture of a talar dome osteochondral lesion.

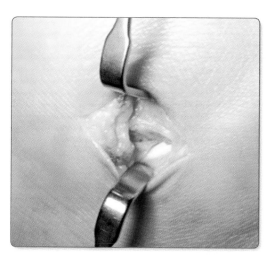

Figure 1.3 Retinaculum incision with exposure of the peroneal tendons.

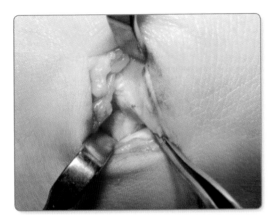

Figure 1.4 The lateral ligaments are exposed below the peroneal tendon.

The calcaneofibular ligament (CFL) is more distinct and is found deep to the peroneal tendons, passing downward and posteriorly towards the peroneal tubercle
- The joint space underneath the fibula must be inspected to ensure that there are no soft tissue entrapments or bony avulsions that should be excised
- The insertion of the ligaments on the distal fibula should be freshened by removing the periosteum of the inner distal fibula with rongeurs
- The ATFL and the CFL are then plicated and reattached to the distal fibula (**Figure 1.5**)

Ligament reattachment
- After preparation of the distal fibula, two suture anchors incorporating a 2-0 nonresorbable suture are inserted into the ATFL and CFL footprints
- The sutures are passed from inside to outside the capsule–ligamentous complex in the direction of the ATFL and CFL, starting distally in order to hitch up the capsule towards the distal fibula
- It is advisable to place a padded kidney dish under the heel on the operating table to raise the talus anteriorly in the ankle mortise before securely tying the suture knots
- As the sutures are tied, beginning with the CFL suture anchor (**Figure 1.6**), the ankle is held by the assistant in dorsiflexion and eversion
- Multiple resorbable vertical mattress sutures can then be placed to reinforce the repair using the free cuff of fibular periosteum

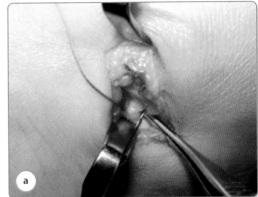

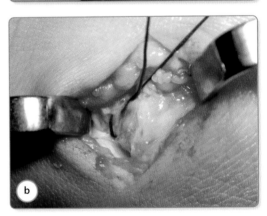

Figure 1.5 Plication of the calcaneofibular and anterior talofibular ligaments and ATFL complex.

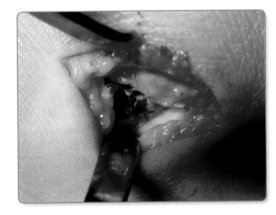

Figure 1.6 Closure with absorbable stitches.

- It is possible to further reinforce the repair by inserting sutures from the fibular periosteum into the inferior extensor retinaculum (Gould modification)

- After the repair the ankle is gently examined for stability using the anterior drawer test and the talar tilt test

Possible perioperative complications

- Division of the lateral branch of the superficial peroneal nerve or the sural nerve must be avoided to avoid pain from a neuroma
- Branches of the lesser saphenous vein are also at risk and sacrifice of small branches may be necessary for access

Closure

- After thorough irrigation with 0.9% saline, the skin incision is sutured (**Figure 1.7**) and Steri-Strips are applied
- A pneumatic ankle brace or a light cast is applied, keeping the ankle in slight dorsiflexion and eversion

Postoperative management

Postoperative regimen

- No weight-bearing is permitted during the first 2 weeks
- 2–6 weeks postoperatively: the ankle is placed in a removable pneumatic walking brace.

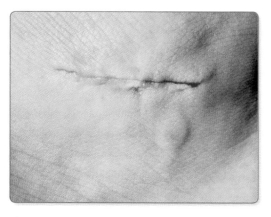

Figure 1.7 Intradermal suture.

The patient can increase their weight bearing and active range of motion exercises of the ankle but must avoid plantarflexion and inversion, which would stretch the repair. Passive stretching is also avoided. Swelling and edema control using an elastic compression stocking, ice, and deep tissue massage should be encouraged

- 6–12 weeks post-operatively: the patient can discontinue use of the pneumatic walker and can be provided with a lace-up ankle brace. Progressive resistive and proprioceptive exercises may be continued during the following 2–4 months
- 3 months postoperatively: running, cutting, and pivoting sports can be resumed. The brace is worn for sports for 6 months

Early-phase complications

- Wound breakdown
- Infection
- Sural nerve injury or neuroma
- Instability or recurrence
- Stiffness and overtightening
- Complex regional pain syndrome

Outpatient follow-up

- Patients are assessed at 6-month intervals for 2 years and then discharged
- Further examinations will be necessary only if symptoms develop again or if a new trauma occurs

Prevention of future injury

- A sport-specific balance training program may be effective for reducing acute-onset injuries in athletes
- A history of previous lateral ankle sprain is associated with an increase in the risk of future sprain of the contralateral ankle. In order to prevent this, prophylactic protection may be helpful: a semi-rigid ankle brace is less expensive than ankle taping and offers similar results
- Postural control and muscle reaction time are fundamental variables that must be considered

Further reading

Colville MR. Surgical treatment of the unstable ankle. J Am Acad Orthop Surg 1998; 6:368–377.

Ferkel RD, Chams RN. Chronic lateral instability: arthroscopic findings and long-term results. Foot Ankle Int 2007; 28:24–31.

Guillo S, Bauer T, Lee JW, et al. Consensus in chronic ankle instability: Aetiology, assessment, surgical indications and place for arthroscopy. Orthop Traumatol Surg Res 2013; 99:S411–9.

Maffulli N, Del Buono A, Maffulli GD, et al. Isolated anterior talofibular ligament Brostrom repair for chronic lateral ankle instability: 9-year follow-up. Am J Sports Med 2013; 41:858–864.

Nery C, Raduan F, Del Buono A, et al. Arthroscopic-assisted Brostrom-Gould for chronic ankle a long-term Follow-up. Am J Sports Med 2011; 39:2381–2388.

Ng ZD, Das De S, Modified Brostrom-Evans-Gould technique for recurrent lateral ankle ligament instability. J Orthop Surg (Hong Kong) 2007; 15:306–310.

Lateral ligament reconstruction with fibular periosteal flap in chronic ankle instability

Indications

Inversion sprains of the ankle are one of the most common injuries in sport. Therefore anterolateral ligament complex injury can occur. In the majority of cases, conservative treatment is effective (Petersen et al, 2013) with a specific rehabilitation program focused on obtaining stability and proprioception to achieve a complete recovery for sporting activity, even with a low grade of ligaments insufficency. Occasionally this injury, especially in the case of ankle sprain, relapses or combines high-grade injuries of anterior talofibular ligament and calcaneofibular ligament and may cause chronic ankle instability. It can cause limitation in sporting activity, functional loss, and eventually can be associated with cartilage damage and chronic synovitis. In these particular settings surgery is the treatment of choice to recreate stability structures. Lateral ligament complex reconstruction is achievable using a fibular periosteal flap: a strong tissue with appropriate mechanical and physical features to reinforce or substitute the floppy or damaged ligaments (Rudert et al, 1997; Benazzo et al, 2013). This surgery is indicated in the following cases:

- Patients with chronic ankle instability due to traumatic anterior talofibular ligament (ATFL) injury associated with thinning or tear of the calcaneofibular ligament (CFL)
- Patients of any age complaining of ankle instability during sport or those with a history of ankle sprain
- Patients with chronic ankle instability despite at least 6 months of rehabilitation, propriocepive activity, and ankle strengthening

Preoperative assessment

Clinical assessment

- Patients report recurring ankle sprain regardless of symptoms
- Patients complain of ankle instability, often associated with pain and swelling
- The examiner assesses for the presence of anterior and lateral laxity with a positive anterior drawer test and talar tilt test
- Clinical assessment also pays attention to the range of motion and clinical signs of synovitis or cartilage damage
- To perform the anterior drawer test the examiner stabilizes the distal leg with the patient seated on the table or supine with the foot over the end of the table. With the other hand, the examiner pulls the foot anteriorly; if there is laxity compared with other side, it reveals a damaged ATFL
- To perform the talar tilt test, the examiner stabilizes the distal leg in a neutral position and inverts the ankle. The examiner then determines how much inversion is present. A positive test is pathognomonic of CFL injury

Imaging assessment

Radiographs

- Anteroposterior and lateral views identify any previous fractures or bony avulsion
- Stress radiographs may detect the ankle laxity grade
- Radiograph identifies signs of impingement or early post-traumatic osteoarthritis, secondary to a chronic instability

Magnetic resonance imaging (MRI)
- MRI identifies ligament injury as thinning and disorganization of fibers or their absence (**Figures 2.1** and **2.2**)

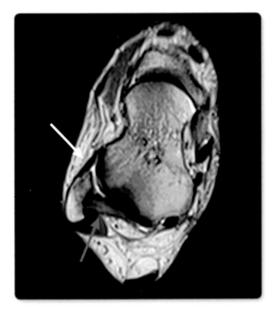

Figure 2.1 T1-weighted axial MRI shows normal anterior talofibular (white arrow) and posterior talofibular (red arrow) ligaments.

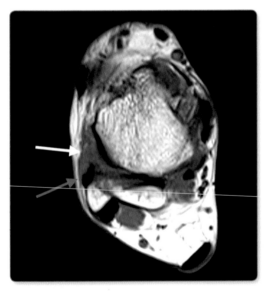

Figure 2.2 T1-weighted axial MRI shows the absence of the anterior talofibular ligament (white arrow). It is possible to identify some residual fibers (red arrow).

- MRI is also useful for detecting associated osteochondral lesions and/or synovitis, and can be helpful in planning an associated surgery
- It confirms the presence of ATFL tear associated with CFL partial injury or tear

Timing of surgery
- Surgery takes place when conservative treatment fails to improve symptoms, after at least six months of specific physiotherapy
- The instability must be assessed objectively, with clinical assessment and imaging
- No edema or any sign of recent sprain should be present at the time of surgery and the ankle must have a complete range of motion
- Acute surgery is possible in selected cases in athletes with MRI findings of ligament injuries associated with capsular laceration, considering also the level of sport and singular functional requests

Surgical preparation
Surgical equipment
- 2.8 mm titanium suture anchors (1 or 2 anchors depending on which ligaments are damaged)

Equipment positioning
- Two surgeons, seated side by side, next to the operated foot

Patient positioning
- Lay the patient supine, with a gel pad under the ipsilateral gluteus, to allow a slight internal rotation of the leg
- A tourniquet is applied to the upper thigh in order to avoid bleeding

Further preparation
- Antibiotic prophylaxis: we use cefazolin 2 g EV, half an hour before the surgery

Surgical technique
Exposure
- Inflate the tourniquet to 320 mmHg
- Make a lateral, curved, L-shaped incision with anterior concavity, from 6 cm proximally over the tip of lateral malleolus ending 3 cm

distally from it (**Figure 2.3**), just posterior to the malleolus, to allow better exposure of the grafting site and of the ankle joint (**Figure 2.4**)

- Check the residual ATFL and CFL ligaments, if present, to evaluate which is to be restored; and so we know if it is necessary to split the periosteal flap or not
- Do not detach residual ligaments if present; use them as a guide to overlap the periosteal neo-ligaments

- Evaluate possible laxity or discontinuity of the capsule (often in acute cases) to suture it

Ligament reconstruction

- After the exposure of the peroneal malleolus, starting from about 5 cm proximal to the malleolar summit, isolate the periosteal flap (**Figure 2.5**), making it as large as possible, especially when splitting of the flap into two is required
- Gently detach the periosteal flap from the bone with a detacher. Do not carve and snap the flap
- Turn the fibular flap and suture it using an absorbable stich to the fibular insertion, in order to avoid tearing when in tension (**Figure 2.6**)
- In the case of splitting of the flap, some sutures are required at the level of the splitting point in order to reinforce the structure and avoid tearing when in tension (**Figure 2.7**)

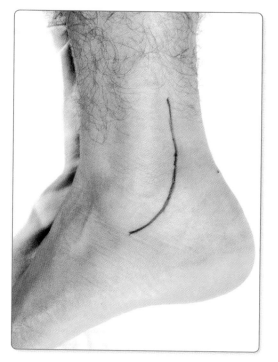

Figure 2.3 Lateral, curved, L-shaped incision.

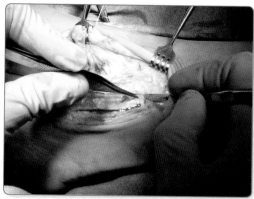

Figure 2.5 Isolate the periosteal flap.

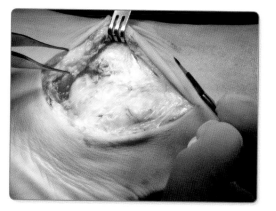

Figure 2.4 Exposure of the lateral ankle joint

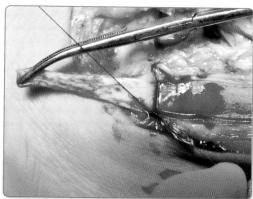

Figure 2.6 Suture the flap's fibular insertion with an absorbable stich, in order to avoid tearing when in tension.

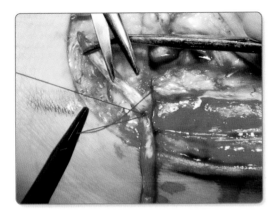

Figure 2.7 Suture the split flap at the base, to reinforce it and avoid tear propagation.

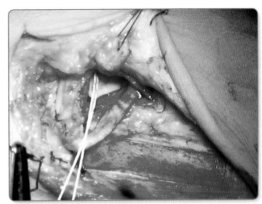

Figure 2.8 Fix the flap at the talus with a 2.8 mm titanium anchor.

- Once the periosteal flap is folded, re-evaluate the length to decide the fixing point to get a neo-ligament with proper tension
- Fix the flap onto the talus at the anatomic AFTL insertion point with a 2.8 mm titanium suture anchor (**Figure 2.8**)
- If the neoligament is long enough, it can be doubled by fixing it to the talus at half its length and then turning the distal half back on the fibula (**Figure 2.9**)
- When a residual ligament is present, it can be overlapped by the periosteal flap, and they can be sutured together with a thin absorbable wire after anchoring the flap at the talus (**Figure 2.10**)
- In both cases the ligament fixation on the talus must be performed with the foot in slight eversion to avoid excessive tension which would cause stiffness
- If the CFL is injured, the periosteal flap must be split in two parts, and the posterior half of doubled flap is fixed onto the calcaneus with an additional 2.8 mm titanium anchor (**Figure 2.11**)

Possible perioperative complications

- Rupture of the flap
- Occurs when the flap is too thin. In this case you have to suture the flap
- Dis-insertion from the fibula: anchor the flap at the fibula with another 2.8 mm anchor. To

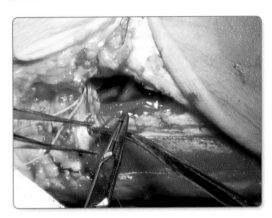

Figure 2.9 The flap length is enough to double it.

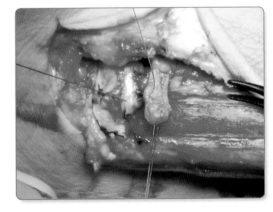

Figure 2.10 Overlap and suture the residual ligament above the neoligament.

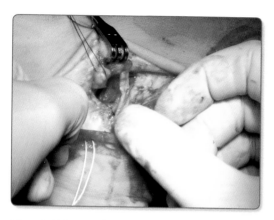

Figure 2.11 in case of a calcaneofibular ligament tear, split the flap and fix the posterior part at the calcaneus.

avoid disinsertion, apply sutures on the basis of the flap

Closure

- Close the subcutaneous and cutaneous layers with standard sutures
- In case of capsular tear, close the tear with absorbable sutures
- Apply one drain proximally to the wound and remove it 24 hours later

Postoperative management

- Place a short fiberglass leg cast to immobilize the ankle for 3 weeks

- Avoid weight bearing for 3 weeks; patients can use crutches
- After 3 weeks place a reinforced fiberglass leg cast (a walker cast) allowing progressive full weight bearing
- After 6 weeks, it is possible to recover the mobility starting passively
- Continue with proprioceptive exercises and ankle strengthening, with isometric contractions first
- Advance with eccentric strengthening exercises from day 65 postoperatively
- Progressively increase the training load, clinically assessing joint stability, swelling, and pain. If everything looks satisfactory, the patient can cautiously start with sport activities, but not before 4 months from surgery

Outpatient follow-up

- Wound evaluations at 7 and 14 days
- Change of plaster cast at 21 days to a full weight-bearing plaster cast
- Remove the second plaster cast after 42 days and assess the stability for permission to start with FKT
- Medications: nonsteroidal anti-inflammatory drugs, if pain is present, and thromboembolism prophylaxis until full weight-bearing is achieved

Further reading

Benazzo F, Zanon G, Marullo M, Rossi SM. Lateral ankle instability in high-demand athletes: reconstruction with fibular periosteal flap. Int Orthop 2013; 37:1839–1844.

Petersen W, Rembitzki IV, Koppenburg AG, et al. Treatment of acute ankle ligament injuries: a systematic review. Arch Orthop Trauma Surg 2013; 133:1129–1141.

Rudert M, Wülker N, Wirth CJ. Reconstruction of the lateral ligaments of the ankle using a regional periosteal flap. J Bone Joint Surg 1997: 79-B:446–451.

3 Lateral ligament stabilization of the ankle: the Williams procedure

Indications

- This is indicated if there have been more than three acute ankle sprains in 6 months, or laxity of the ankle along with a feeling of instability
- Failure of conservative treatment, which includes mechanical bracing of the ankle, and various techniques of physiotherapy for at least 6 months, may lead to surgical treatment
- The Williams procedure may be performed for mechanical or functional instability

Preoperative assessment

Clinical assessment

- Clinical assessment includes differentiation between instability and pain. Pain may not necessarily be associated with the unstable ankle; therefore other causes of ankle pain should be excluded
- The clinical examination includes routine range of motion measurements of the ankle, subtalar, and midfoot region
- Muscle force evaluation primarily involves the peroneal muscles. Weakness of these may be a cause of ankle instability
- Specific tests include drawer test examination of the ankle and evaluation of proprioception using a modified Romberg test. The patient should also be assessed for joint hyperlaxity

Imaging assessment

- In order to assess mechanical instability of the ankle a routine stress radiograph of both ankles should be taken for every patient
- The criteria for mechanical instability are:
  - A 6° (or greater) difference between the injured ankle and the uninjured ankle in the lateral tilt of the talus; and
  - A difference of 2 mm in the posterior opening of the tibiotalar joint between the injured ankle and the uninjured ankle

Timing for surgery

- After failure of conservative treatment, operative treatment is indicated

Surgical preparation

Surgical equipment

- Chlorhexidine skin preparation
- Pneumatic thigh tourniquet
- Sterile adhesive exclusion drapes
- Knife handle and size 10 and 15 blades
- Self-retaining retractor
- Dissecting scissors
- Needle holders
- Size 0 Vicryl sutures
- Forceps
- Size 4-0 Vicryl Rapide

Equipment positioning

- Following the skin incision the self-retaining retractor is placed within the wound to reveal the underlying lateral capsuloligamentous complex

Patient positioning

- The patient lies supine with the thigh and buttock elevated on a pillow to enable ease of approach to the anterolateral side of the ankle
- An ankle block procedure with local anesthesia can be administered in a day care facility

Surgical technique

Exposure

- A lateral oblique approach immediately anterior to the fibula is used. The skin is exposed dorsally to the long extensors
- Care must be taken not to harm the branch of the superficial peroneal nerve (**Figure 3.1**). The fat of the sinus tarsi is exposed and lifted dorsally until the extensor retinaculum is exposed

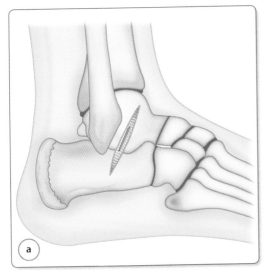 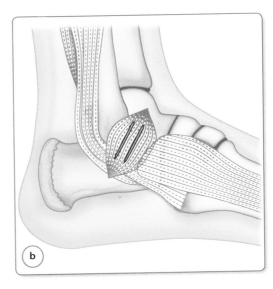

Figure 3.1 (a) Surgical approach – skin incision. (b) Proximal and distal cuts in the capsule.

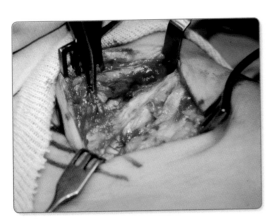

Figure 3.2 Proximal cut in the capsule.

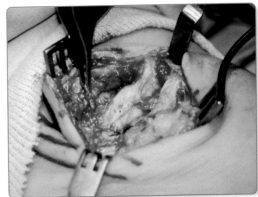

Figure 3.3 Distal cut in the capsule: base of the extensor digitorum brevis fascia.

- Two parallel cuts are made in the capsuloligamentous complex. One is a 2–3 mm cut anterior to the fibula including the ankle joint capsule until the lateral side of the ankle joint is exposed. A plantar incision stops at the peroneal muscles and care must be taken not to harm the peroneal tendons
- The peroneal tendon sheath is usually opened at this stage in order to verify that the tendons are intact, and appropriate care is taken to prevent damage to the tendons (**Figure 3.2**). Another cut parallel to the first (about 1.5 cm distally to

the first one) is made at the base of the extensor digitorum brevis (EDB) at the beginning of the fascia of the EDB, thus creating a soft tissue bridge over the lateral side of the talus consisting of the extensor retinaculum, the remnants of the anterior talofibular ligament, and the joint capsule (**Figure 3.3**)

Ligament reconstruction

- At least five Vicryl (no. 0) sutures are passed from the anterior edge of the fibula to the fascia of the EDB and back towards the anterior fibular joint capsule under the soft tissue bridge in a U-shape, putting the hindfoot in eversion and tying the sutures under tension. This causes approximation of the EDB fascia to the anterior ankle joint capsule under the soft tissue bridge, with stabilization of the ankle joint (**Figure 3.4**)

- At this stage anterior–posterior stability should be checked and the range of ankle motion should be assessed to ensure that the ligaments are not too tight. Another four sutures are needed, two from the bridge to the anterior side of the fibula, and two to the side of the EDB with Vicryl no. 0 sutures securing the soft tissue bridge with the extensor retinaculum, to the reconstructed ligaments

(**Figure 3.5**)
- The soft tissue bridge is sutured to the capsule to create tension in the repair (**Figure 3.6**)
- The incision is closed using nylon 4-0 or Vicryl Rapide 4-0
- The ankle is secured in a U-shaped cast splint

Possible perioperative complications

- Immediate postoperative risks include the usual postoperative complications such as infection, nerve damage, mainly to the dorsal branch of the superficial peroneal nerve, and limited ankle motion due to overtightening of the ligaments

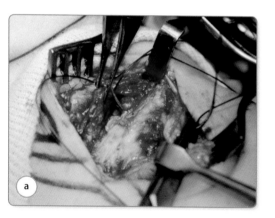 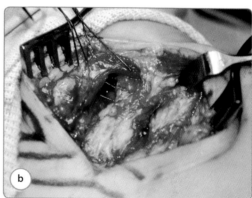

Figure 3.4 (a-b) Passing sutures from the anterior area of the fibular capsule under the bridge and back to the anterior area.

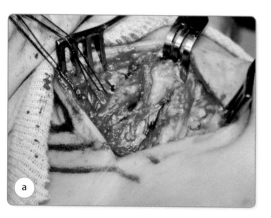 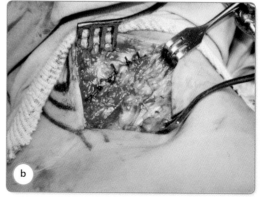

Figure 3.5 (a-b) Tensioning and tying the sutures under the bridge.

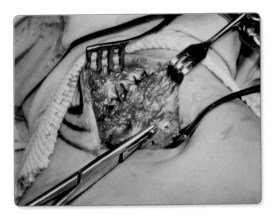

Figure 3.6 Securing the bridge to the capsule.

Postoperative management

- The leg is kept in a nonweight bearing U-shaped splint for 2 weeks. This is followed by full weight-bearing walking in an ankle brace for 6 weeks
- Physiotherapy commences 2 weeks after the operation and first includes range of motion exercises of the ankle, followed by strengthening of the muscles around the ankle, and finally proprioception exercises of the ankle

Outpatient follow-up

- After 2 weeks the patient returns for follow-up to remove the cast and commence weight bearing and physiotherapy. In 6–8 weeks the patient is ready to engage in sports activities

Further reading

Mann G, London E, Chaimsky G, Nyska M. The Williams procedure. In: Mann G, Nyska M (eds), The unstable ankle. Human Kinetics, 2002.

Anatomic deltoid ligament repair

Indications

- Eversion ankle sprains with consequent medial instability. This type of injury may cause a partial or complete deltoid ligament tear; however surgery is rarely needed to ease healing of an isolated deltoid ligament rupture
- Lateral malleolar injuries with talar shift in the ankle mortise suggesting a bimalleolar equivalent injury. When the mortise remains wide medially after anatomic reduction of the fibular fracture, exploration of the medial side is warranted to address entrapment of the torn deltoid ligament
- Disruption of the distal tibiofibular syndesmosis. In this situation it is sometimes desirable to repair the deltoid and in doing so impart additional stability to a syndesmotic reconstruction, particularly in the athlete
- Late-stage adult acquired flat foot deformity. Repair of the chronically deficient deltoid ligament may be required when there is abnormal tilt of the talus in the ankle mortise
- In the setting of the soft tissue balancing required during total ankle replacement surgery

Mechanism of injury and classifications

The most characteristic injury patterns are:

- Pronation–abduction, pronation–external rotation, or supination–external rotation injuries of the ankle (Lauge–Hansen classification)
- Danis–Weber B and C fibular fractures
- Syndesmotic sprains
- Both a medial fracture and deltoid ligament injury; medial injury combinations include (Pankovich et al, 1979):
  - Rupture of the deep and superficial deltoid
  - Fracture of the anterior coliculus
  - Fracture of the anterior colliculus and the deep deltoid
  - Fracture of the posterior colliculus
  - Supracollicular fracture
- Avulsion or chip fractures
- Deltoid ligament incompetence after medial malleolar fixation (Tornetta, 2000)

Preoperative assessment

Clinical assessment

Physical examination

- Deltoid ligament injuries cause pain, tenderness, swelling, and bruising on the medial side of the ankle (**Figure 4.1**)
- It is important to evaluate the syndesmosis for a sprain and the fibula for the presence of fracture
- The syndesmosis is examined for injury using a combination of palpation and stress tests. If there is an obvious syndesmosis injury of fibular fracture, do not proceed to perform stress tests. Tenderness will be evident with palpation over the anterior-inferior tibiofibular ligament and pain will be appreciated during

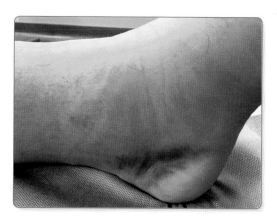

Figure 4.1 Medial side edema.

external rotation and dorsiflexion of the ankle against the articular facet of the fibula. The external rotation stress test also helps evaluate the integrity of the deltoid ligament
- As the superficial component of the deltoid ligament crosses and stabilizes the subtalar joint, clinical evaluation of subtalar stability against valgus heel stress is required
- If a fibular fracture is present, the medial side of the ankle must be assessed for the presence of a bimalleolar equivalent injury
- Pressure on the proximal portion of the fibula assesses the presence of a Maisonneuve fracture and hence the likelihood of syndesmotic and deltoid ligament disruption

Imaging assessment

Radiographs
- Standard plain radiographs include anteroposterior, mortise, and lateral views of the ankle
- Radiographic signs of a syndesmosis injury and hence deltoid injury include:
  - *Increased medial clear space between the medial malleolus and talar body*: this is assessed on a true mortise view. Any asymmetry between the medial and lateral clear spaces around the talar body may be pathologic. The usual range of clear space is 3–5 mm but identifying asymmetry is more important than taking measurements
  - *Decreased tibiofibular overlap*: this is measured as the distance between the medial border of the fibula and the most lateral point of the posterior arm of the incisura fibularis. The radiographic value decreases with internal rotation of the ankle (normal value >6 mm or >42% of the width of the fibula on the anteroposterior view or >1 mm on the mortise view)
  - Syndesmosis and deltoid injuries are also suggested by more than 1 mm lateral subluxation of the talus or obvious talar tilt on the mortise view (Porter et al., 2014)
- It is important to remember that isolated deltoid rupture does not necessarily involve a widening of the medial clear space as the lateral malleolus holds the talus in position; evidence of this type of injury may be difficult if only static radiographs are used. Gravity stress lateral radiographs or eversion stress

radiographs may be useful to detect subtle syndesmotic and deltoid injuries
- When a proximal fibular fracture is suspected, anteroposterior and lateral radiographs of the entire fibula must be taken

Computed tomography (CT)
- CT may detect minimal (2–3 mm) syndesmotic diastasis that is not visible on plain radiographs

Magnetic resonance imaging (MRI)
- MRI is highly sensitive and specific for the diagnosis of syndesmotic and deltoid injuries
- It has been demonstrated that the widening of the medial tibiotalar clear space on the mortise view may not be closely associated with deep deltoid ligament injuries. For these reasons, MRI may be helpful to allow appropriate and early diagnosis, as well as prevention of chronic medial instability, ostheoarthritis, and medial ankle impingement syndrome (Chabra, 2010) (**Figures 4.2** and **4.3**)

Timing of surgery
- Surgical delay should be minimized to that which permits soft tissue swelling to subside

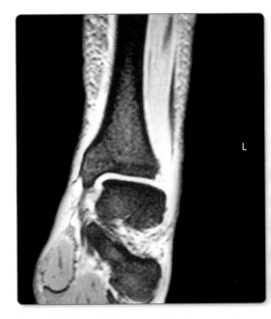

Figure 4.2 MRI: deltoid ligament dislocated under the medial malleolus, showing high signal in the deltoid with fibers in the medial gutter.

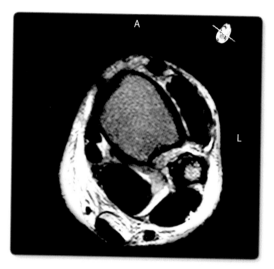

Figure 4.3 MRI: syndesmotic lesion with the fibula lying outside the syndesmosis.

- It is advisable to undertake a closed reduction and casting of a severely swollen subluxed ankle to allow soft tissue recovery before performing surgery on both sides of the ankle

Surgical preparation

Special surgical considerations

- Restoring stability to the ankle is dependent on a perfect reduction of any fibular fracture with restoration of the talar alignment and symmetric radiographic clear spaces. For this reason, commence the surgery on the lateral side of the ankle as it may not be necessary to proceed to deltoid repair in the acute situation. Obviously if there is a medial malleolar fracture this needs reduction and fixation

- After fibular fracture fixation, the syndesmosis requires evaluation in the usual way with external rotation stress radiographs of a fibular hook test under fluoroscopic control. If the lateral side of the ankle is stable, again it is not always necessary to repair the deltoid ligament as it will heal by scarring. A medial repair is indicated if the medial tissue are introflected in the medial gutter
- For patients with chronic instability it may be desirable to arthroscopically assess the ankle first. In this way the syndesmosis can be assessed for injury and the medial gutter tested for stability by assessing the clear space available for introduction of the arthroscope (Hintermann et al., 2002)
- Hintermann medial instability classification:
  - *Grade 1*: Stable – it is difficult to part the tibiotalar joint space by more than 2 mm
  - *Grade 2*: Moderately unstable – the surgeon is able to introduce a 5 mm arthroscope into the medial gutter
  - *Grade 3*: Severely unstable – it is possible to see to the back of the ankle with a large arthroscope if traction is used

Surgical equipment (Figure 4.4)

- Needle holder
- Sutures
- Scalpels, blades no. 11 and 21
- Forceps: toothed tissue forceps, Adson's tissue forceps, Kocher's, Kelly's and mosquito forceps
- Scissors
- Luer bone rongeur
- Retractors: Farabeuf and Mathieu
- Hohmann bone elevators
- Bone curettes
- Mallet
- Osteotome

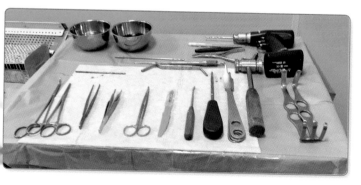

Figure 4.4 Surgical equipment.

- Drill equipment: hand drill, drill guide, and drill bits
- Kirschner (K)-wires
- Screws
- Screwdriver

Equipment positioning

- The surgical equipment is positioned near the surgeon, on the side of the ankle that is to be operated

Patient positioning

- The patient lies in the supine position
- A tourniquet is placed on the thigh
- The stability of the syndesmosis is tested with external rotation and abduction stress under fluoroscopy
- At the appropriate time the limb is exsanguinated and tourniquet inflated

Further preparation

- The patient receives a single dose of prophylactic intravenous antibiotics at induction of anesthesia
- It is preferable to perform the procedure under general anesthetic but regional blocks can be utilized

Surgical technique

Lateral approach for the stabilization of the syndesmosis

- Make a direct lateral approach to the fibula at the level of the syndesmosis, with a 4–6 cm skin incision (**Figure 4.5**)

- Be careful not to damage the sural nerve. The diastasis must be reduced, correcting the malrotation
- The fibula is anatomically reduced and the syndesmosis may be stabilized with two fully threaded position screws across four cortices (**Figure 4.6**)
- After the syndesmosis reduction it is possible to repair the anterior inferior tibiofibular ligament with suture anchors, although it usually heals successfully by scarring in the acute situation without primary repair

Medial approach for repair of the deltoid ligament

- Make a 4–6 cm curvilinear incision, distally and parallel to the medial malleolus (**Figure 4.7**)
- It is possible to find the deltoid ligament within the medial gutter of the ankle, preventing talar reduction, especially when there is a fibular fracture or syndesmosis injury
- After the exposure, evaluate the deltoid ligament status. If the deep component is compromised in conjunction with a syndesmotic injury, an early repair of the ligament can be performed
- Reflect the posterior tibialis tendon (PTT) sheath longitudinally off the back of the medial malleolus, allowing improved exposure and inspection of the articular surfaces. Any cartilage injury can then be debrided and drilled if necessary
- No. 1 Vicryl sutures are placed through both the deep and the superficial components of the

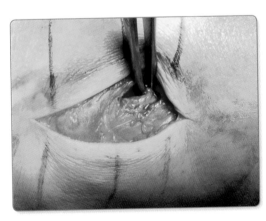

Figure 4.5 Lateral incision for syndesmotic repair.

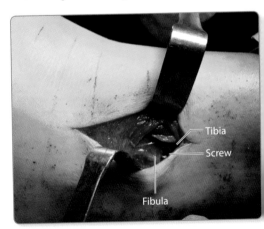

Figure 4.6 Lateral side after reduction with screws.

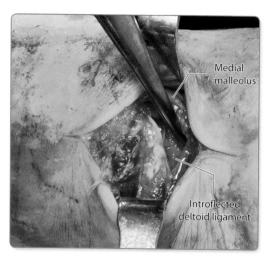

Figure 4.7 Medial side incision below the medial malleolus.

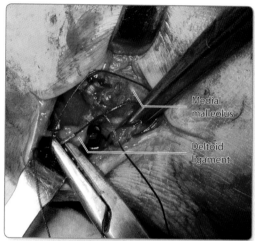

Figure 4.8 Deltoid ligament detached from the medial malleolus: medial repair with absorbable sutures.

deltoid ligament (**Figure 4.8**). The deep fibers are sutured and tied before the placement of the superficial sutures. The deltoid sutures should be secured only after the osteosynthesis is completed and a definitive fixation on the lateral side is obtained, in order to protect the deltoid repair
- The final result, including joint reduction and alignment of the talus, may be evaluated with fluoroscopy before starting the skin closure

Possible perioperative complications

- Section of the lateral branch of the superficial peroneal nerve or sural nerve: isolate every structure that must be protected and remain aware of the position of the tibial neurovascular bundle

Closure

- After thorough irrigation with 0.9% saline, the skin incisions are sutured and Steri-Strips are applied
- A pneumatic ankle brace or a light cast is applied
- An elastic bandage can be applied over the skin to avoid distal edema
- Radiographic assessment is performed to check final alignment (**Figure 4.9**)

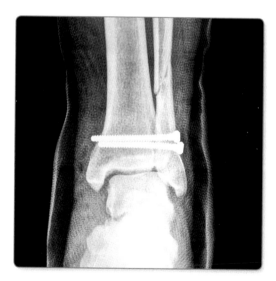

Figure 4.9 Radiograph showing anatomic alignment after surgery.

Postoperative management

Postoperative regimen

- 0–3 weeks postoperatively: immobilization is recommended in a nonweight-bearing boot
- 3–6 weeks postoperatively: gentle range of motion recovery is achieved, the patient is still encouraged to wear a nonweight-bearing boot

- 6 weeks postoperatively: the patient may begin weight bearing in a hinged ankle brace
- 9 weeks postoperatively: the patient may start running, always wearing an ankle brace or supportive taping
- 12 weeks postoperatively: the patient can stop using joint protection

Postoperative complications

- Infection
- Wound breakdown
- Stiffness

- Complex regional pain syndrome (CPRS)
- Osteoarthritis
- Instability or recurrence

Outpatient follow-up

- Patients are assessed at 6-month intervals for 2 years and then discharged
- Further examinations will be necessary only if symptoms develop again or if new trauma occurs

Further reading

Bhadra AK, Porter DA. Tibiofibular syndesmosis reduction and fixation. In: Kitakoa HB (ed.), Master techniques in orthopaedic surgery – the foot and the ankle, 3rd edn. Philadelphia: Lippincott, Williams & Wilkins 2013: 479–494.

Chhabra A, Subhawong TK, Carrino JA. MR imaging of deltoid ligament pathologic findings and associated impingement syndromes. Radiographics 2010; 30:751–761.

Hintermann B, Boss A, Shäfer D. Arthroscopic findings in patients with chronic ankle instability. Am J Sports Med 2002; 30:402–409.

Lynch SA Assessment of the injured ankle in the athlete. J Athl Train 2002; 37:406–412.

Pankovich AM, Sivaram MS. Anatomical basis of variability in injuries of the medial malleolus and the deltoid ligament. II. Clinical studies. Acta Orthop Scand 1979; 50:225–236.

Porter DA, Jaggers RR, Barnes AF, et al. Optimal management of ankle syndesmosis injuries. Open Access J Sports Med 2014; 5:173–182.

Tornetta P 3rd. Competence of the deltoid ligament in bimalleolar ankle fractures after medial malleolar fixation. J Bone Joint Surg 2000; 82: 843–848.

Indications

The spring or calcaneo-navicular complex ligament is classically described with three bundles. The superomedial calcaneonavicular ligament (SMCNL), or the ligamentum neglectum, and the inferior calcaneonavicular ligament, or the true spring ligament. The third ligament was identified under the cartilage covering the spring ligament fibrocartilage complex.

The role of the spring ligament complex and the tibialis posterior tendon is to maintain the integrity of the longitudinal arch of the foot.

The indications for spring ligament reconstruction are:

- Acquired adult flat foot deformity caused by tibialis posterior tendon dysfunction (TPTD)
- Tibialis posterior tendon tear with spring ligament tear
- Isolated spring ligament tear

Preoperative assessment

Clinical presentation

- Patients either present with an acute injury following trauma or a more chronic history in the case of TPTD
- They often have pain and swelling over the medial hindfoot, exacerbated by activitiy
- There may be a history of progressive medial arch collapse or rarely acute flat foot deformity

Clinical assessment

- Examination can demonstrate a flat foot with a valgus heel and forefoot abduction
- Look for swelling and tenderness localized over the posterior tibial tendon and around the medial and plantar aspects of the talonavicular joint
- Specific tests for TPTD are inability to perform a single-limb heel rise with weakness of the tibialis posterior muscle

- The ankle, subtalar, and midfoot motion should be assessed to exclude degenerative changes in these joints

Imaging assessment

Radiographs

- A standard weight-bearing, anteroposterior radiograph of the foot can show uncovering of the talonavicular joint
- A lateral radiograph may demonstrate lowering of the arch in the talonavicular area and loss of calcaneal pitch

Ultrasonography

- Ultrasonography is useful to assess the tibialis posterior tendon and can reveal tears as well as thickening and synovitis
- Assessment of spring ligament tears using ultrasonography is, however, difficult and MRI is the imaging of choice to confirm a tear

Timing for surgery

- A spring ligament tear with associated complete tear of the tibialis posterior tendon is an indication for immediate repair
- With a collapsed arch with tendon pathology, treatment is initially conservative for at least 6 months. This includes orthotics, anti-inflammatories, and physical therapy

Surgical preparation

Surgical equipment

- 2.0 mm drill bit
- 4.5 mm drill bit
- FiberTape (Arthrex, Inc., Naples, FL)
- SutureLasso (Arthrex, Inc., Naples, FL)
- Tendon shuttle (Arthrex, Inc., Naples, FL)
- Bioabsorbable 3.5 mm BioComposite SwiveLock (Arthrex, Inc., Naples, FL)
- Biotenodesis screws 4.75 mm
- Suture Ethibond no. 5 (Ethicon, Inc., a division of Johnson & Johnson, Somerville, NJ)

Patient positioning

- The patient is positioned supine with the knee extended and a lateral support
- The foot must be slightly rotated externally
- A tourniquet is applied to the thigh

Further preparation

- Prophylactic antibiotics are indicated as per local guidelines
- The tourniquet is inflated to 100 mmHg above systolic blood pressure prior to the surgical incision

Surgical technique

Exposure

- The exposure extends from the posterior aspect of the medial malleolus along the tibialis posterior tendon to the medial navicular tuberosity and distal to it for about 1–2 cm
- The posterior aspect of the tibialis posterior tendon sheath is carefully opened
- A synovectomy is performed in case of synovitis
- Excision of the tendon is performed if there is a degenerative tendon, leaving a distal stump for a tendon transfer
- The talonavicular joint and the spring ligament are now visible for evaluation

Ligament evaluation

- When the spring ligament is completely torn, the head of the talus is exposed during forefoot abduction (**Figure 5.1**)

- In case of spring ligament attenuation, the head of the talus is mildly protruded and seen throughout the incompetent attenuated ligament
- The tear in the spring ligament is usually vertical in the area of the superomedial band of the ligament
- The margins of the tear are debrided to refresh the edges prior to reconstruction

Ligament reconstruction

Navicular preparation

- The first stage consists of dissection of the navicular bone to expose the dorsal and plantar surfaces of the medial tuberosity. A 4.5 mm vertical tunnel is then drilled through the medial tuberosity

Sustentaculum tali preparation

- The second stage is exposure of the posterior sustentaculum tali and detachment of the flexor hallucis longus (FHL) tendon sheath posterior to it. This helps protect the neurovascular bundle, which lies just posterior to it. A 2 mm tunnel is drilled horizontally in the sustentaculum tali from anterior to posterior, protecting the FHL and neurovascular bundle throughout

Ligament preparation

- The third stage is direct suturing of the spring ligament with Ethibond to strengthen the remnant of the ligament (**Figure 5.2**)
- The fourth stage is reconstruction of the ligament to increase the strength of the

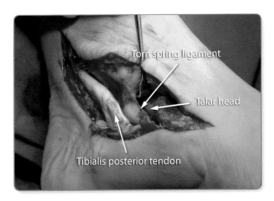

Figure 5.1 Torn spring ligament with tibialis posterior tendon insufficiency.

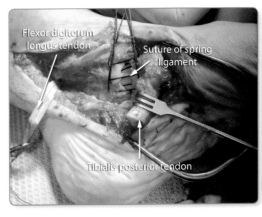

Figure 5.2 Direct spring ligament suture.

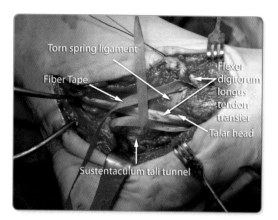

Figure 5.3 FiberTape reconstruction.

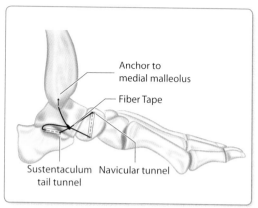

Figure 5.4 Final spring ligament reconstruction.

medial structures using FiberTape. This is passed through the tunnel with SutureLassos in a figure of 8 (**Figure 5.3**).

Final tensioning

- The fifth step is to tighten the direct sutures of the spring ligament while the foot is stressed into adduction
- This is followed by tightening of the figure of eight FiberTape with the foot in the same position
- The remnants of the suture tape are anchored with the bioabsorbable 3.5 mm BioComposite SwiveLock to the medial malleolus for anatomic reconstruction of the anterior part of the deltoid ligament
- A medially displaced varizing calcaneal osteotomy is now performed to correct the valgus of the heel as a regular procedure for flat foot reconstruction (**Figure 5.4**)

Possible perioperative complications

- Complications during surgery generally occur during the sustentalum tali drilling
- There is a risk of drill penetration into the joint as well as fracture of the sustentaculum
- The neurovascular bundle is also extremely close to the posterior aspect and should be protected behind the sheath of the FHL

Closure

- The peritenon is closed with absorbable suture
- No drains are needed
- Subcutaneous tissue and skin are closed in a standard fashion

Postoperative management

- A postoperative nonweight-bearing below-knee cast is applied for 6 weeks
- During the initial 3 weeks the foot is held in plantarflexion and inversion to unload the reconstruction
- For the following 3 weeks the foot is maintained in a plantigrade position
- After 6 weeks the cast is removed and full weight bearing begins, protected by an ankle brace with intensive physical therapy aimed at improving inversion strength

Outpatient follow-up

- The first visit is at 3 weeks postoperatively, to change the cast position from an inverted plantar-flexed foot into a plantigrade foot position
- At the second visit, after 6 weeks, the cast is removed and full weight bearing with an ankle brace commenced. Physiotherapy can also commence at this stage, aiming for full range of motion at 3 months

Further reading

Palmanovich E, Shabat S, Brin YS, et al. Anatomic reconstruction technique for a plantar calcaneonavicular (spring) ligament tear. J Foot Ankle Surg 2015 [Epub ahead of print].

Taniguchi A, Tanaka Y, Takakura Y, et al. Anatomy of the spring ligament. J Bone Joint Surg Am 2003; 85:2174–2178.

Tryfonidis M, Jackson W, Mansour R, et al. Acquired adult flat foot due to isolated plantar calcaneonavicular (spring) ligament insufficiency with a normal tibialis posterior tendon. Foot Ankle Surg 2008; 14:89–95.

6 Open reduction and internal fixation of lateral malleolar fractures

Indications

- Displacement of greater than 2 mm, especially in young athletes with high functional demand
- Fractures associated with rotation and/or shortening of the lateral malleolus

Preoperative assessment

Clinical assessment

- On inspection, the ankle may appear swollen and/or deformed. Associated ecchymosis, blistering, and open wounds may be found
- Assess for tenderness along the distal fibula and the medial malleolus
- The swelling and pain found are likely to limit movement
- Significant distortion of the patient's anatomic profile suggests the joint is also subluxed or even dislocated
- Assess the distal neurovascular status by examining the patient's cutaneous sensation in the distribution of the peripheral nerves supplying the foot and ankle, in addition to checking for pedal pulses. If swelling precludes accurate assessment of the patient's vascularity, capillary refill, pulse oximetry, and hand-held Doppler ultrasonography help to distinguish between a perfused and nonperfused limb

Imaging assessment

Radiographs

- Standard lateral and mortise radiographs are recommended (oblique view with the foot internally rotated 20° to bring the lateral malleolus into the same coronal plane as the medial malleolus during imaging) (**Figure 6.1**)

Computed tomography (CT)

- In cases associated with intra-articular involvement of the tibial plafond, CT is recommended
- CT can also be used where the diagnosis is in doubt

Timing for surgery

- Immediate reduction of a dislocated or subluxed ankle in association with a fracture is recommended to avoid further soft tissue swelling and cartilage injury. The ankle should be immobilized with either a backslab plaster or a spanning external fixator, prior to definitive fixation
- Significant soft tissue damage resulting in blisters require a temporary spanning external fixator, with the joint appropriately aligned and soft tissues protected. This should be done in conjunction with elevation and application

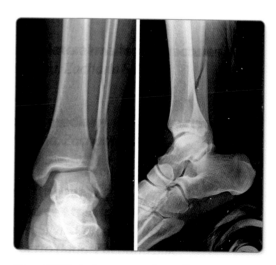

Figure 6.1 Fibular fracture: mortise and lateral radiographic view.

of ice to assist in reducing the level of tissue swelling prior to definitive surgery
- A delay to surgery is advised until the soft tissue envelope has recovered, as evidenced by the resolution of blisters, epithelialization of abrasions, and presence of the 'wrinkle sign' around the operative site

Surgical preparation

Surgical equipment
- A selection of reduction forceps, along with a system of plates and screws of 3.5 mm diameter with the option of anatomically contoured locking plates, should be available. In the majority of cases, one-third tubular plates used in conjunction with lag screw fixation will suffice

Equipment positioning
- Position the image intensifier on the opposite side of the operative site. Place the screen near to the foot end of the bed

Patient positioning
- The patient is positioned supine on a radiolucent operating table with a sandbag under the ipsilateral hip to aid in internally rotating the ankle
- A tourniquet can be applied to the upper thigh
- The contralateral limb can be positioned with the hip flexed and the leg elevated on a support

Further preparation
- Perioperative antibiotic prophylaxis
- Lateral and mortise views with fluoroscopy before surgery

Surgical technique

Exposure
- Direct access using a lateral skin incision, between the anterior compartment muscles, innervated by the deep peroneal nerve, and the lateral compartment muscles, innervated by the superficial peroneal nerve
- Take care to avoid an overly anterior incision to help avoid accidental injury to the superficial peroneal nerve, which provides sensation to the dorsolateral aspect of the foot at this level.

Occasionally, it is injured depending on the pathologic anatomy of the fracture; therefore careful preoperative documentation of the neurovascular status is mandatory. Injury to this nerve can cause a painful neuroma with dysesthetic symptoms
- If preferred, a dorsolateral incision may be utilized to apply a posterior fibular plate, as well as providing access to reduce a posterior malleolar fracture. In this case, the incision runs between the Achilles tendon and the peroneal tendons; careful dissection is necessary to avoid injury to the sural nerve

Fracture reduction
- Accurate reduction requires restoration of the exact length and rotation of the distal fragment. If unsure, a useful measure is the talocrural angle, which is subtended between a line perpendicular to the distal plafond and a line running between the tips of both malleoli. The normal angle is approximately $83° ± 4°$. Use of image intensifier on the opposite ankle is suggested to compare the restoration of fibular length if it is in doubt
- An anatomic reduction is most easily observed after careful exposure of the fracture site before reduction. A useful check is to specifically check the posterior fibular cortex is in correct alignment
- Once fibular length and rotation has been restored, attempt to temporarily stabilize the fracture with pointed reduction forceps until definitive fixation is achieved (**Figure 6.2**)

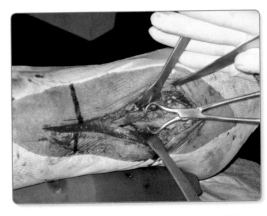

Figure 6.2 Temporary stabilization of the reduced fibular fracture with the aid of pointed reduction forceps.

Implant positioning

- If an anatomic reduction is achieved, absolute stability can be provided by the insertion of one or two lag screws, providing compression at the fracture site. Small-fragment 3.5 or 2.7 mm screws may be used, or in case of compromised bone quality 2.4 mm screws may be utilized
- The technique of lag screw fixation involves drilling a hole in the near cortex of a diameter equal to that of the screw's thread diameter (**Figure 6.3**); following this a drill guide is advanced into the first hole to allow accurate placement of the second hole in the far cortex, which should be of a diameter equal

to the core diameter of the screw (**Figure 6.4**). Measure the appropriate length using a depth gauge, tap the hole (if required), and insert a fully threaded cortical screw (**Figure 6.5**)
- In most cases, the direction of this screw can be perpendicular to the fracture
- Following stabilization with a lag screw, the fracture must be protected with a neutralization plate, such as a one-third tubular plate (**Figure 6.6**)
- If anatomic reduction cannot be achieved, fibular locking plates increase strength and allow for stable fixation with only two screws in the distal or proximal fragment
- If the fracture pattern is such that posterior

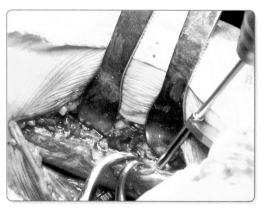

Figure 6.3 Lag screw technique: first hole in the near cortex, with a thread diameter of the selected screw.

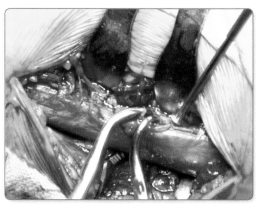

Figure 6.5 Lag screw technique: stabilization of the reduction with the screw to provide compression at the fracture site.

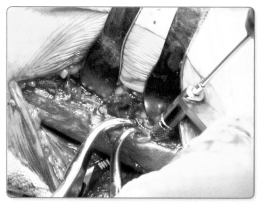

Figure 6.4 Lag screw technique: second hole in the far cortex using a drill guide to maintain direction. The hole drilled is equal to the core diameter of the selected screw.

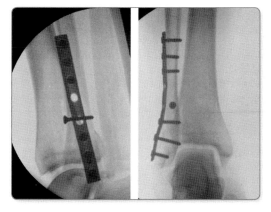

Figure 6.6 Lag screw and one-third tubular plate correctly placed: fluoroscopy showing anteroposterior and lateral views.

displacement is a risk, a posterior antiglide plate may be an appropriate solution
- While anatomic locking plates are slightly more prominent than one-third tubular plates, they are very helpful in elderly patients with osteoporosis, in cases where the distal fragment is too small to accommodate at least two screws, and in cases with extended comminution
- In this last case the minimally invasive plate osteosynthesis (MIPO) technique is employed, which involves sliding the plate under the skin, thereby respecting the soft tissue envelope around the fracture site. Indirect reduction techniques are used to restore length and rotation under fluoroscopic control. Axial alignment is restored using the anatomically contoured plate (**Figure 6.7**)

Possible perioperative complications

- Injury to the superficial peroneal nerve
- Injury to the sural nerve
- Fracture displacement
- Infection and/or wound breakdown

Closure

- Close the fascia and subcutaneous tissues with absorbable sutures
- Close the skin with nonabsorbable suture

Postoperative management

- Nonsteroidal anti-inflammatory drugs
- Prevention of venous thromboembolism, if required
- Nonweight bearing for 6 weeks
- Elevate limb in a cast for 2 weeks
- Postoperative lateral and mortise radiographs

Outpatient follow-up

- Day 14: remove the sutures; remove the plaster cast; begin ankle mobilization exercises without weight bearing
- Week 6–8: repeat ankle radiographs and initiate partial weight bearing if radiographs are satisfactory
- Week 12: full weight bearing is permitted

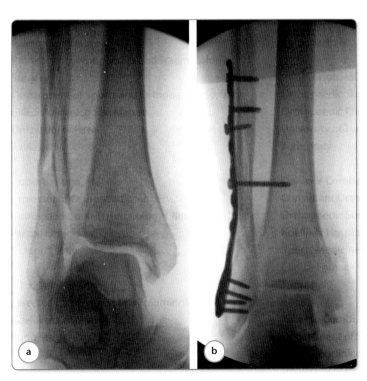

Figure 6.7 Comminuted metaphyseal fibular fracture (a); the fracture was reduced and stabilized by an anatomic plate, inserted using a minimally invasive plate osteosynthesis technique. The locking screws allowed this plate to be used like an internal–external fixator (b).

a

b

Implant removal

- Occasionally, the plate or screws can lie prominently, especially if the patient has limited adipose tissue. After the fracture has united, the plate can be removed if it is believed to be causing the patient discomfort
- A posterior plate may irritate the overlying peroneal tendons, leading to tendonitis and/or even rupture. In this case, the plate can also be removed pre-emptively once union has occurred

Further reading

Hahn DM, Colton CL. Malleoli. In: AO Principles of Fracture Management, 2nd edn. Ruedi TP, Buckley RE, Moran CG (ed.). New York; Thieme Verlag, 2007: 871–897.

Messmer P, Perren SM, Suhm N. Screws. In: AO Principles of Fracture Management, 2nd edn. Ruedi TP, Buckley RE, Moran CG (ed.). New York; Thieme Verlag, 2007: 213–225.

Ostrum RF. Posterior plating of displaced Weber B fibula fractures. J Orthop Trauma 1996;10:199–203.

Sommer C, Schutz M, Wagner M. Internal fixator. In: AO Principles of Fracture Management, 2nd edn. Ruedi TP, Buckley RE, Moran CG (ed.). New York; Thieme Verlag, 2007: 321–335.

Open reduction and internal fixation of medial malleolar fractures

Indications

- A displaced fracture of greater than 2 mm of translation is an indication for surgery
- In young athletes with high functional demands, inferior translation can be a sufficient condition to justify surgical treatment

Preoperative assessment

Clinical assessment

Basic signs

- On examination, the ankle may appear swollen and bruised with a distortion in the normal anatomic profile of the ankle joint. Note of any blisters and open wounds overlying the fracture. Palpation of the medial malleolus will reveal tenderness
- Swelling and pain limit the range of motion
- Document the neurovascular status of the foot prior to surgical intervention

Imaging assessment

Radiographs

- Lateral and mortise radiographs of the ankle are standard. A mortise view is obtained by internally rotating the leg by 15–20° so that the X-ray beam is nearly perpendicular to the intermalleolar line (**Figure 7.1**)

Computed tomography (CT)

- CT may be performed if the diagnosis is in doubt or if there is an associated fracture of the tibial plafond

Timing for surgery

- Immediate reduction of a dislocated or the subluxed ankle in association with a fracture is recommended to avoid further soft tissue swelling and cartilage injury. The ankle should be immobilized with either a backslab plaster or a spanning external fixator, prior to definitive fixation
- Significant soft tissue damage resulting in blisters requires a temporary spanning

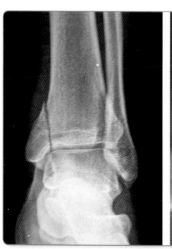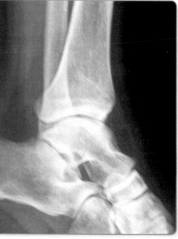

Figure 7.1 Mortise and lateral radiographic views identifying a medial malleolar fracture.

external fixator, with the joint appropriately aligned and soft tissues protected. This should be done in conjunction with elevation and application of ice to assist in reducing the level of tissue swelling prior to definitive surgery
- A delay to surgery is advised until the soft tissue envelope has recovered, as evidenced by the resolution of blisters, epithelialization of abrasions, and presence of the 'wrinkle sign' around the operative site

Surgical preparation

Surgical equipment
- Kirschner (K) wires, cannulated or noncannulated partially threaded cancellous screws, pointed reduction forceps, 3.5 mm cortical screws, and wires for tension band wiring

Equipment positioning
- Position the image intensifier on the opposite side of the operative site. Place the screen near to the foot end of the bed

Patient positioning
- The patient is positioned supine on a radiolucent operating table
- A tourniquet can be applied to the upper thigh
- The contralateral limb may be positioned with the hip flexed and the leg elevated on a support (**Figure 7.2**)

Further preparation
- Perioperative antibiotic prophylaxis
- Lateral and mortise views with fluoroscopy before surgery

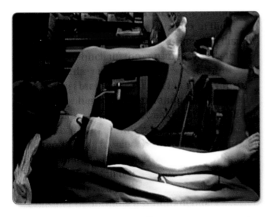

Figure 7.2 Patient positioning allowing easy access to the medial malleolus.

Surgical technique

Exposure
- The medial malleolus is approached using either a straight or posteriorly curved medial incision, partly depending on the need to avoid compromised skin
- Take particular care not to damage the saphenous nerve and/or the long saphenous vein, which both run in the subcutaneous tissue, anteriorly and superiorly to the medial malleolus

Fracture reduction
- After exposure of the fractured medial malleolus, the fracture site is cleared of debris and periosteum to avoid inadvertent interposition that may hinder an anatomic reduction
- Accurate restoration of the fragment is required, paying special attention to any abnormality of rotation
- Pointed reduction forceps may be used to obtain temporary stabilization
- The fracture may be stabilized with two K-wires prior to surgical fixation

Implant positioning
- Two partially threaded 4 mm screws are inserted perpendicular to the fracture under fluoroscopic guidance to achieve compression (**Figure 7.3**)
- If the fragment is too small to insert two screws, it is possible to use one screw in conjunction with a K- wire or a polylactic acid (PLLA) rod to provide resistance against rotation of the fragment (**Figures 7.4** and **7.5**)
- Another option in difficult cases is use of a tension band wiring technique to reduce and stabilize the fracture using a metal wire diameter ranging from 1 to 1.8 mm, passing through a proximal tibial anchor point created using either a 3.5 mm hole or a screw (**Figures 7.6** and **7.7**)

Possible perioperative complications
- Injury of the long saphenous vein and/or the saphenous nerve anteriorly. Posteriorly, the posterior tibial artery and tibial nerve are in close proximity

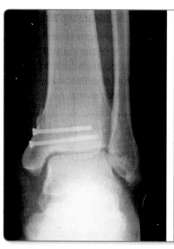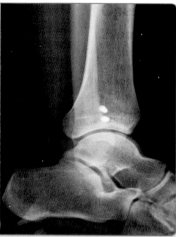

Figure 7.3 Postoperative radiographs of a fracture that was reduced and stabilized with two screws.

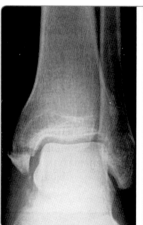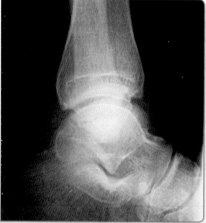

Figure 7.4 Anteroposterior and lateral radiographic views of a small tibial malleolar fracture.

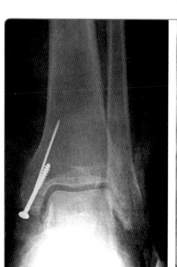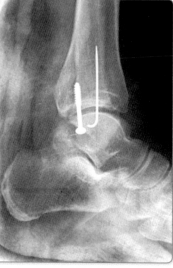

Figure 7.5 Postoperative radiographs following fixation of a medial malleolar fracture with one screw and one K-wire.

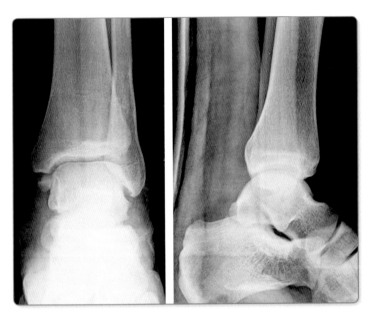

Figure 7.6 Anteroposterior and lateral radiographic views of a small and fragmented medial malleolar fracture.

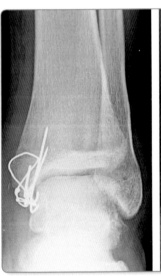
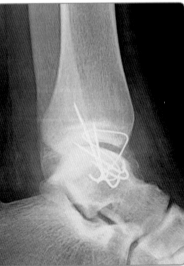

Figure 7.7 Post-operative radiographs of a medial malleolar fracture fixed using a tension band wire.

- Fracture redisplacement, non-union and delayed union

Closure

- No drainage is needed
- Close the fascia and subcutaneous tissues with absorbable sutures
- Close the skin with nonabsorbable suture

Postoperative management

- Nonsteroidal anti-inflammatory drugs
- Prevention of venous thromboembolism, if required
- Nonweight bearing for 6 weeks
- Elevation of limb in a cast for 2 weeks

- Postoperative lateral and mortise radiographs

Outpatient follow-up

- Day 14: remove the sutures, remove the plaster cast, and begin ankle mobilization exercises without weight bearing

- Weeks 6–8: repeat ankle radiographs and initiate partial weight bearing if radiographs are satisfactory
- Week 12: full weight bearing is permitted

Implant removal

- Screws and metal cerclage wires that are superficial can be painful. If so, these can be removed after the fracture has united

Further reading

Hahn DM, Colton CL. Malleoli. In: AO Principles of Fracture Management, 2nd edn. Ruedi TP, Buckley RE, Moran CG (ed.). New York; Thieme Verlag 2007:871–897.

Schepers T, De Vries MR, Van Lieshout EM, et al. The timing of ankle fracture surgery and the effect on infectious complications; a case series and systematic review of the literature. Int Orthop 2013; 37: 489–494.

Tarkin IS, Sop A, Pape HC. High-energy foot and ankle trauma: Principles for formulating an individualized care plan. Foot Ankle Clin N Am 2008; 13:705–723.

Walling AK, Sanders RW. Ankle fractures. In: Surgery of the foot and ankle, 8th edition. Coughlin MJ, Mann RA, Saltzman CL (ed.). Philadelphia; Mosby Elsevier, 2007:1973–2016.

Treatment of osteochondral lesions of the talus using 'one-step' bone marrow-derived cell transplantation

Indications

The current indication for this procedure is a chronic type 2 osteochondral lesion of the talar dome that is less than 1.5 cm^2 in area and less than 5 mm deep (Giannini et al, 2005).

- It is best reserved in patients below the age of 50 years due to the greater intrinsic regenerative potential
- Early degree of arthritis
- The treatment is not recommended for patients with advanced osteoarthritis, kissing lesions of the ankle, rheumatoid arthritis, or severe malalignment or laxity unless already adequately treated

Preoperative assessment

Clinical assessment

- The symptoms associated with chronic osteochondral lesions include a mild, and sometimes continuous, pain that is usually associated with physical activity
- Asymptomatic cases are not uncommon
- Walking on uneven ground may increase the patient's symptoms
- Swelling, stiffness, weakness, and reduced range of motion may also be present, especially with degenerated osteochondral lesions
- Patients may complain about the inability to load the joint and, in the presence of loose bodies, they may also experience catching, locking, or clicking
- Palpation often evokes tenderness on the posteromedial or anterolateral aspect of the talus
- The anterior drawer and talar tilt tests should be performed to exclude associated ligament injuries as high-grade sprains are usually found in association with osteochondral lesions

Imaging assessment

Radiographs

- While routine radiographs of the ankle may miss a proportion of small osteochondral lesions of the talus, it is still necessary to help detect associated pathologies such as joint misalignment, anterior impingement, and foot deformities
- Standard anteroposterior and medial-lateral views of the ankle joint may help identify a large detached fragment, especially in acute cases (Navid and Myerson, 2002)

Computed tomography (CT)

- CT is a valuable investigation in the workup of such patients as it can identify subchondral bone pathology or cysts
- The main benefit is that it can clearly delineate the size, shape, extent, and localization of any bony lesions, if present (Ferkel et al, 1991)

Magnetic resonance imaging (MRI)

- MRI remains the gold standard investigation for the diagnosis of osteochondral lesions, providing information about edema, cartilage status, and the soft tissue envelope
- The sensitivity of MRI is high when correlated to arthroscopic findings (81–83% or even higher) (Bae et al, 2012)
- The most frequent signs suggestive of an osteochondral lesion are a decreased signal intensity on T1-weighted images and increased signal intensity on T2-weighted images

- In cases where the fragment remains partly tethered to the underlying bone, there is less correlation between what is observed at the time of arthroscopy and the preoperative T2-weighted MRI (Bae et al, 2012)

Timing for surgery

- Low grades of osteochondral lesions are scarcely symptomatic and patients may be either misdiagnosed or initially treated nonoperatively, taking care to follow the patient up over time
- Large lesions are usually painful and scarcely respond to a nonoperative treatment alone
- Once the lesion is diagnosed, the patient may undergo surgery

Surgical preparation

Surgical equipment

- Platelet-rich fibrin kit
- Cell harvesting and concentration equipment
- Arthroscopic equipment:
  - 8 mm and 11 mm diameter stainless steel arthroscopic cannulas with a window on one side. These should be specifically designed to allow the surgeon to slide a scaffold (either collagen or hyaluronic) impregnated with bone marrow-derived cells directly to the site of the lesion
- A flat tip probe to help manipulate the scaffold into the lesion

Platelet-rich fibrin production

- Platelet-rich fibrin is produced using an automated system either on the day of or the day before the planned operation
- The procedure involves harvesting 120 mL of venous blood with a 16G needle connected to a sterile container previously prepared with an anticoagulant solution
- The container is then placed inside the Vivostat System and processed by centrifuge
- At the end of the cycle, a syringe containing approximately 6 mL of platelet-rich fibrin is extracted and either used immediately or stored at –35°C for later use
- If the extract is frozen, the platelet-rich plasma fibrin must be gradually warmed to room temperature 30 minutes prior to its intended use

Patient positioning

- Set up the patient in the prone position using either spinal or general anesthesia and prepare a sterile surgical field
- The anatomic landmarks for this procedure are the posterior superior iliac spine and iliac crest

Surgical technique

Harvesting of bone marrow-derived cells

- A dedicated kit for osteochondral regeneration, developed by Novagenit (Mezzolombardo, Trento, IT), contains all the equipment required for the bone marrow harvesting, concentration, and implantation
- Insert an 11G needle to a depth of approximately 3 cm into the iliac crest and aspirate a total of 60 mL of bone marrow (**Figure 8.1**)
- This is placed in a bag preloaded with 500 units of heparin mixed with 10 mL of a 0.9% saline solution
- Bone marrow harvesting takes place step by step by inserting the needle into different locations on the iliac crest to maximize the collection of stromal cells useful for cartilage regeneration and minimize dilution of the sample from aspiration of peripheral blood

Preparation of bone marrow-derived cell concentrate

- The 60 mL of bone marrow aspirate to be processed (the minimum amount required by the manufacturer) is injected into the posterior portion of the double-chamber device
- The harvested bone marrow is reduced in volume directly in the operating room by removing most of the red cells and plasma
- After two cycles of centrifugation, the mononuclear cells remaining at the bottom of the anterior chamber are aspirated with a syringe to obtain 6 mL of cell concentrate

Implantation of bone marrow-derived cells

Exposure

- Standard anteromedial and anterolateral arthroscopic portals are created with the patient now in a supine position

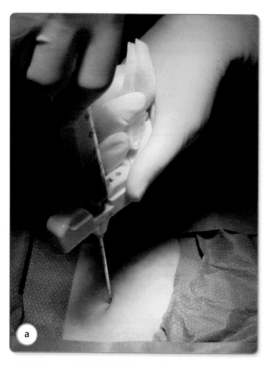

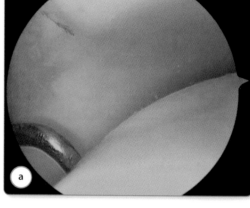

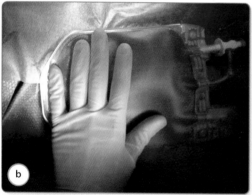

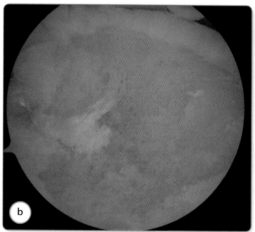

Figure 8.1 (a) Bone marrow is aspirated by inserting an 11G needle to a depth of approximately 3 cm into the iliac crest. (b) A total of 60 mL of bone marrow is harvested from subsequent aspirations.

Figure 8.2 (a) The osteochondral lesion is located. (b) Debridement of the lesion until the healthy bleeding bone is seen.

- The tourniquet is inflated to 280 mmHg after exsanguination of the limb
- The osteochondral lesion is identified (**Figure 8.2a**) and prepared by debriding the detached cartilage and subchondral bone until the healthy bleeding bone is reached (**Figure 8.2b**)
- Using a calibrated probe, the lesion size is measured. The scaffold is cut to an

appropriate size and shape and loaded by capillary action with 2 mL of bone marrow concentrate (**Figure 8.3**)

Implant positioning

- The large diameter cannula is inserted through the arthroscopic portal closest to the lesion

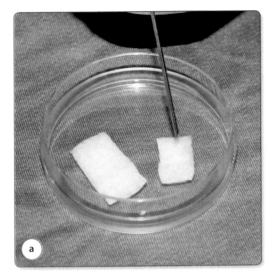

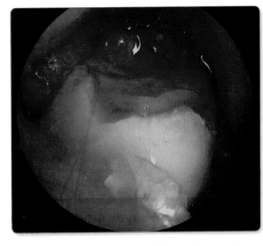

Figure 8.4 The composite is carefully placed into the lesion site using a flattened probe.

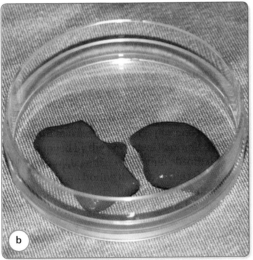

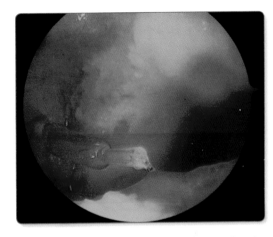

Figure 8.3 (a) The scaffold is cut to match an appropriately measured size and shape. (b) The scaffold is ready to be loaded by capillary action using 2 mL of bone marrow concentrate.

Figure 8.5 A layer of platelet-rich fibrin gel is spread on the implant to provide an additional supply of growth factors.

- The prepared composite is fed through the cannula up to the margin of the lesion
- When the cannula is removed, the composite is carefully placed into the debrided lesion using a flattened probe (**Figure 8.4**)
- A layer of the harvested platelet-rich fibrin gel is then finally spread on the implant to provide an additional supply of growth factors (**Figure 8.5**)

Possible perioperative complications

Surgical complications sustained during or after this procedure are very rare, occurring in less than 1% of cases. These include:

- Injury to blood vessels and/or nerves
- Intra-articular breakage of surgical instruments

Closure

- Skin closure may be achieved using absorbable 3-0 sutures, using a single interrupted stitch for each portal
- Standard dressings and an elastic bandage are then used

Postoperative management

- Patients are usually discharged on the day of or the day after surgery
- Continuous passive motion is performed on the day after surgery and gradually increased as tolerated
- During the first 6 weeks postoperatively, walking is permitted using two crutches and with no weight bearing on the affected side. After the first 6 weeks, progressive weight bearing can be permitted, gradually increasing the load the patient is able to sustain over the next 2–4 weeks
- Low-impact sports such as swimming and cycling are permitted 4 months postoperatively
- High-impact sports such as tennis, soccer, and running can resume at about 8–10 months

Early postoperative complications

- Infection
- Phlebitis
- Swelling

Outpatient follow-up

- Clinical evaluation at 1, 2 and 4 months postoperatively is initially recommended, followed by semi-annual clinical, radiologic and MRI follow-up for 2 years

Further reading

Bae S, Lee HK, Lee K, et al. Comparison of arthroscopic and magnetic resonance imaging findings in osteochondral lesions of the talus. Foot Ankle Int 2012; 33:1058–1062.

Ferkel RD, Flannigan BD, Elkins BS. Magnetic resonance imaging of the foot and ankle: correlation of normal anatomy with pathologic conditions. Foot Ankle 1991; 11:289–305.

Giannini S, Buda R, Faldini C, et al. Surgical treatment of osteochondral lesions of the talus in young active patients. J Bone Joint Surg Am 2005; 87:28–41.

Navid DO, Myerson MS. Approach alternatives for treatment of osteochondral lesions of the talus. Foot Ankle Clin 2002; 7:635–649.

Arthroscopic treatment of osteochondral lesions of the talus

Indications

The arthroscopic treatment of osteochondral lesion of the talus (OLT) is indicated in:

- Symptomatic unstable OLT, regardless of age
- Symptomatic stable OLT in younger patients (<30 years) to prevent further degenerative changes to the chondral surfaces
- Large lesions (>2 cm²)
- Symptomatic OLT in patients older than 30 years, when the conservative options (cast immobilization, bracing, physical therapy, anti-inflammatory drugs) have failed to relieve all the symptoms
- Symptomatic OLT when a concomitant surgical procedure is necessary for chronic instability

Preoperative assessment

Clinical assessment

- Symptomatic patients with OLT often complain of ankle pain as well as instability. These symptoms are exacerbated by activity. Locking and catching may indicate the presence of a displaced fragment
- Physical examination of a symptomatic OLT may reveal medial, central, or lateral joint line pain. There may also be evidence of a joint effusion and loss of ankle range of movement
- Evaluation of lateral and anterior–posterior ankle stability (comparing with the opposite side) is essential to confirm or exclude a concomitant chronic instability (**Figure 9.1**)

Imaging assessment

Radiographs

- Weight bearing anteroposterior and lateral views often reveal the larger lesions, but the small to medium defects are difficult to visualize on simple radiographs (**Figure 9.2**)

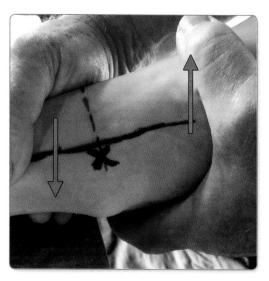

Figure 9.1 Clinical evaluation of ankle stability (lateral and anterior–posterior).

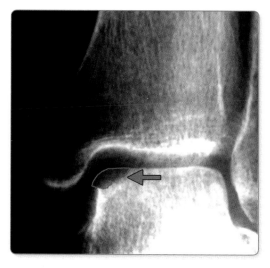

Figure 9.2 Anteroposterior radiograph: a medial osteochondral lesion of the talus (arrow).

Computed tomography (CT)

- CT can assess size and location of the bony part of the lesion
- A three-dimensional reformat image may be useful to evaluate the shape and the orientation of a displaced osteochondral fragment

Magnetic resonance imaging (MRI)

- MRI is useful in detecting more details on soft tissue (cartilage or ligaments injuries) and bone bruises, but the high sensitivity may lead to an overestimation of the bone damage (**Figure 9.3**)

Timing for surgery

- Initial conservative treatment of a symptomatic OLT of a small size (<1 cm^2) should be recommended
- Acute or subacute larger lesions (>2 cm^2) with a displaced fragment should be fixed when following accurate planning of the procedure (i.e. decide if the fragment should be fixed with pins or screws, retrograde or anterograde, open or arthroscopic, etc.)
- Symptomatic OLT should be treated in combination with ligament repair surgery in cases of post-traumatic chronic instability

Surgical preparation

Surgical equipment

- The set for arthroscopic treatment of OLT includes:
  - 4.0 mm 30° arthroscope
  - Invasive or noninvasive distraction device
  - Spinal needle
  - Shaver with 3.5–4 mm blade
  - Angled curette (**Figure 9.4**)
  - Microfracture awl set (angled from 30° to 90°)
  - Absorbable or metallic pins or screws (if fragment fixation is needed)
  - Complete arthroscopic set (a pump is not routinely used)

Equipment positioning

- The arthroscopic tower faces the surgeon on the opposite side of the table, at the patient's shoulder level

Patient positioning

- The patient is placed in a supine position with the foot at the distal end of the table, allowing the surgeon to fully dorsiflex and extend the ankle
- A tourniquet is placed around the upper thigh

Further preparation

- Antibiotic prophylaxis is recommended
- Inflation of the tourniquet (to around 300 mmHg)

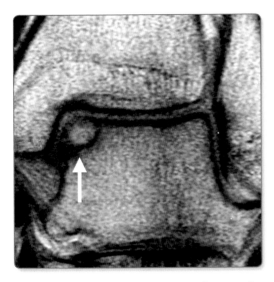

Figure 9.3 MRI: a large bone bruising area adjacent to the osteochondral lesion of the talus.

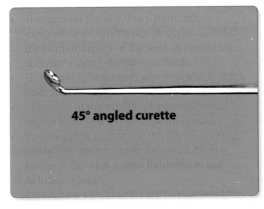

45° angled curette

Figure 9.4 An angled (45°) curette may be useful for the debriding the lesion.

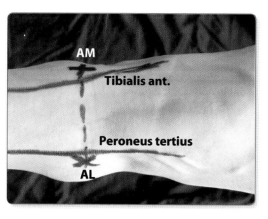

Figure 9.5 Two standard ankle portals: anteromedial (AM) and anterolateral (AL).

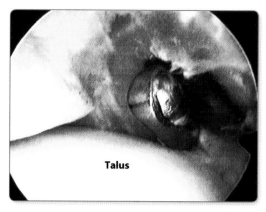

Figure 9.6 Use a shaver to remove the hypertrophic soft tissue.

Surgical technique

Portals

- Two standard ankle portals: anteromedial and anterolateral (**Figure 9.5**)
- Anteromedial portal: 5–7 mm skin incision with a no. 11 blade, just medial to the tibialis anterior tendon, at the level of the joint line
- Use a hemostat for a blunt dissection of the subcutaneous tissue
- Introduce the scope with the ankle maximally dorsiflexed
- Open the water inflow
- Introduce a spinal needle into the anterolateral portal, just lateral to the peroneus tertius tendon, at the level of the joint line
- Check the needle position with a scope view
- Make an anterolateral 5–7 mm skin incision at the spinal needle site. Establish the portal with blunt dissection using a hemostat

Debridement

- In cases with hypertrophic synovial tissue use the shaver to partially remove it, achieving a clear visualization of the OLT (**Figure 9.6**)
- Identify and locate the OLT, palpating the chondral surface with the probe
- Debride the OLT with the shaver, removing the unstable cartilage and the subchondral necrotic bone (**Figure 9.7**)
- Switching the instruments between the portals allows for a more accurate debridement

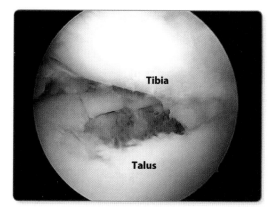

Figure 9.7 Remove the unstable cartilage and necrotic subchondral bone.

Microfracture

- Use a microfracture awl with an angled tip (30°, 45°, 60°, or 90°) and pierce the subchondral plate, making several holes at 3 mm intervals (**Figure 9.8**)
- Avoid creating loose bony fragments during the bone marrow stimulation technique
- The more angled awl (90°) is helpful to treat the posterior part of the OLT

Fragment fixation

- In case of an acute large (>2 cm^2) fragment with its relevant bone portion, which can be partially or totally displaced, consider the fixation options (absorbable or metallic pins, screw)

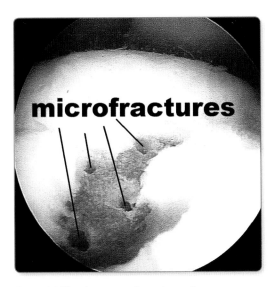

Figure 9.8 Microfractures at 3 mm intervals.

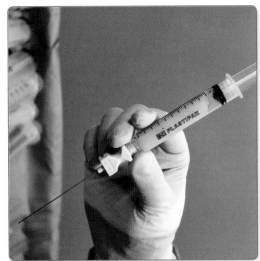

Figure 9.9 Healing enhancement: injecting mesenchymal stem cells from adipose tissue.

- If you choose an arthroscopic fixation, use a spinal needle to find the right fixation angle from an additional medial or lateral access
- Maintain the fragment reduction during the fixation procedure with the probe or a spinal needle
- Convert to an open procedure if necessary to achieve a more stable fixation

Healing enhancement

- Biologic additional procedures may be effective to enhance the cartilage healing: PRP (platelet rich plasma) and MSCs (mesenchymal stem cells) are most commonly used
- PRP:
  - Draw the patient's blood before the surgical procedure
  - Centrifugation is carried out during the arthroscopy
  - At the end of the arthroscopic procedure remove all water from the joint
  - Inject PRP at the OLT site (better under a direct scope view)
- MSCs:
  - Harvest MSCs from the patient's bone marrow (tibia or iliac crest) or adipose tissue (liposuction from the abdomen)
  - MSCs are isolated and concentrated during arthroscopy
  - At the end of the arthroscopic procedure remove all water from the joint
  - Inject MSCs at the OLT site (better under a direct scope view) (**Figure 9.9**)

Possible perioperative complications

- Narrow joint space: use a distraction device
- OLT extends too far posteriorly: make a posterolateral portal
- Bony fragments during debridement: remove these
- Difficulty during an arthroscopic fixation procedure on a large bony fragment: convert to open surgery

Closure

- Close the skin at the portals
- No drain is required
- Simple dressing and a light elastic compression bandage are applied

Postoperative management

- Medications: analgesia, nonsteroidal anti-inflammatory drugs, deep venous thrombosis prophylaxis for 2 weeks

- If the fragment has not been fixed, partial weight bearing for 2 weeks (crutches)
- No weight bearing for 6 weeks in case of fragment fixation

- Immediate mobilization and muscular rehabilitation
- Control radiographs at 2 weeks and 6 weeks in case of fragment fixation

Further reading

McGahan PJ, Pinney SJ. Current concept review: osteochondral lesions of the talus. Foot Ankle Int 2010; 31: 90–101.

Zengerink M, Struijs PAA, Tol JL, van Dijk CN. Treatment of osteochondral lesions of the talus: a systematic review. Knee Surg Sports Traumatol Arthrosc 2010; 18:238–246.

Indications

The indications for an isolated subtalar joint (SJ) arthrodesis include:

- Post-traumatic arthritis
- Inflammatory arthritis
- Coalition of the SJ, with or without a deformity

Severe deformity secondary to a flat foot or cavus varus foot is generally treated with extended arthrodesis (i.e., triple arthrodesis)

Contraindications

- General contraindication include acute or chronic infection or poor vascular status
- A relative contraindication is poor skin quality of the lateral region of the foot but this can be overcome if the medial soft tissues are amenable to a medial approach to the SJ

Preoperative assessment

Clinical assessment

- Clinical examination starts by observing the patient in the standing position. Look at hindfoot alignment, particularly assessing active varus hindfoot movement with tip toe standing, which can be lost with subtalar pathology
- The SJ maybe stiff: check active and passive subtalar movement with the patient in either a prone or a sitting position. This movement also relies on an intact midtarsal joint (Chopart) so this must be assessed at the same time
- There may be swelling and pain in the lateral aspect of the joint at the sinus tarsi and under the tip of the lateral malleolus

Imaging assessment

Radiographs

- Weight-bearing plain radiographs with lateral, anteroposterior, and oblique views are necessary to identify the SJ
- A bilateral anteroposterior view of the ankle is recommended when assessing the position of the ankle, to get a bilateral view of the tibiotalar joint with anteroposterior weight-bearing projection

Computed tomography (CT)

- CT is useful for visualizing bone defects and deformity of the joint:
  - Scans in the coronal plane are the best for visualizing medial talocalcaneal osseous coalitions, pathology involving the lateral process of the talus, and deformity of the talar body
  - Sagittal planes show the posterior SJ and calcaneal body

Magnetic resonance imaging (MRI)

- MRI may detect osteochondral lesions, synovitis with cysts in the posterior space or in the sinus tarsi, as well as bone edema as a sign of chondromalacia of the SJ
- Fibrous and chondral coalitions are best visualized with MRI

Timing for surgery

- Surgery is only indicated after failure of conservative treatment such as:
  - Orthotics and shoe modifications, which may relieve symptoms. The aim is to stabilize the hindfoot with a heel cup moulded orthotic
  - Injection of corticosteroid into the sinus tarsi, which can be both diagnostic and therapeutic

Surgical preparation

Surgical equipment

- 6.5–7.2 mm double or partially threaded screws
- A small joint distractor or laminar spreader
- Ostotomes and chisels
- Power burr
- Kirschner (K)-wires

Equipment positioning

- A C-arm, or preferably a C-arm low dose fluoroscopy, is placed on the same side as the foot to be operated on
- The surgeon stands or sits at the lateral side of the foot, the assistant at the end of the operating table, and a second assistant on the opposite side of the foot to maintain the leg in an internally rotated position

Patient positioning

- The patient is placed in a supine position with a wedge under the ipsilateral hip so that the toes point to the ceiling
- A tourniquet in placed at the upper thigh
- The leg is prepared and draped up to the knee to visualize the long axis of the tibia and the patella, in order to control the correct position of SJ fusion
- It is possible to use a large foam block to lift the leg from the operating table for 360° access to the foot (**Figure 10.1**)
- The iliac crest is prepared just in case a large amount of autologous bone graft is needed

Surgical technique

Exposure

- A longitudinal 7 cm skin incision is made starting under the tip of the lateral malleolus and heading towards the base of the fourth metatarsal. The incision stops at the level of the muscle bell of the extensor digitorum brevis (**Figure 10.2**)

- Care must be taken to prepare the skin flap to avoid postsurgical necrosis of the wound edge. This is a potential complication, especially with poor subcutaneous tissue
- The traditional Ollier oblique incision is avoided because it does not allow extension to the midfoot and it is more likely to injure the lateral branches of the peroneal and sural nerves
- A vertical incision in the retinaculm extensor is made to access the sinus tarsi (**Figure 10.3**)
- All soft tissue is removed and the capsule of posterior SJ is opened
- Articular cartilage or fibrous post-traumatic tissue is resected from joint surface with the aid of a chisel (**Figure 10.4**)
- The whole of the nonarticular surface of the sinus tarsi is decorticated and can be later packed with graft material to aid fusion

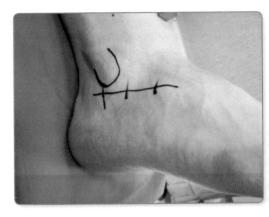

Figure 10.2 Lateral longitudinal approach to subtalar joint.

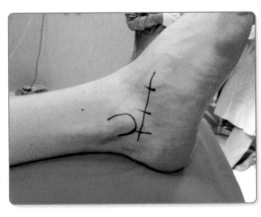

Figure 10.1 The foot is prepped on a foam leg holder.

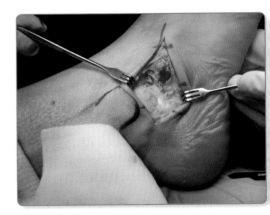

Figure 10.3 View of lateral extensor retinaculum and soft tissue of the sinus tarsi.

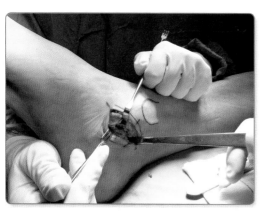

Figure 10.4 Posterior subtalar joint is opened and debrided.

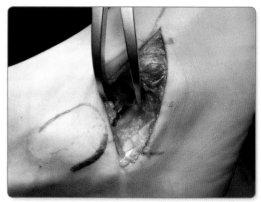

Figure 10.5 A toothed laminar spreader is inserted in the sinus tarsi to gain access to the posterior facet of subtalar joint.

- Care should be taken to remove excessive bone that will disrupt the articular relationship of the SJ. The anterior facet of SJ is then denuded of articular cartilage. A spreader–distractor will help to visualize the posterior SJ (**Figure 10.5**)
- Drilling of the denuded surface, where possible, will help with the fusion. The heel is manipulated to easily obtain the correct axis of the rear foot

Implant positioning

- Once the SJ is aligned it can be temporarily fixed with one or more K-wires
- Definitive fixation is achieved by drilling one or two screws from heel to talus. The first is directed to the talus neck (**Figure 10.6**). It is possible to check the correct direction by visualizing the screw at the bottom of the sinus tarsi. A second screw is directed to the talar body
- Checks on the screw positions are made during the procedure with a fluoroscan. The aim is to obtain a rigid fixation with the correct hindfoot alignment
- Bone graft can be harvested from the lateral wall of the calcaneus. Allograft bone is placed into the gaps in the SJ and the sinus tarsi is packed with bone chips to improve fusion (**Figure 10.7**)

Possible perioperative complications

- Care must be taken not to injure the sural nerve or the superficial branch of the peroneal nerve

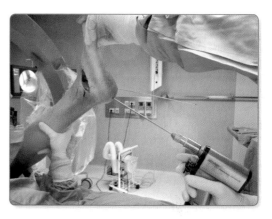

Figure 10.6 A cannulated screw is inserted over a guide pin from the heel directed dorsally into the talus.

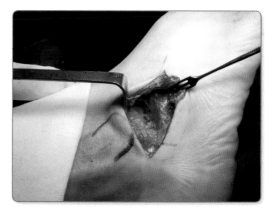

Figure 10.7 Cancellous chips bone graft filled the sinus tarsi at the end of the procedure.

- An axial incision course parallel to the sural and intermediate dorsal cutaneous nerves makes damage less likely
- The direction and length of the screws must be checked to ensure they do not create impingement of the tibiotalar joint or impinge into the subcutaneous heel fat tissue

Closure

- Subcutaneous and skin closure with a 3–0 braided adsorbable inverted suture and skin is closed with a single 4–0 subcuticular absorbable suture
- A drain is used routinely
- A short leg synthetic cast is placed from the anterior tibial tuberosity to half way from the toes

Postoperative management

- The patient is kept nonweight bearing and prescibed antithrombotic prophylaxis

Further reading

Kitaoka HB. The foot and ankle: master techniques in orthopaedic surgery, 3rd edn. Philadelphia: Lippincot Williams & Wilkins, 2013.

Outpatient follow-up

- Starting from 6 weeks the splint is temporarily removed to mobilize the tibiotalar joint
- A compressive short leg sock is advised (18 mmHg pressure) to control the lymphedema
- Active nonweight-bearing mobilization, until 8 weeks is recommended. Patients should avoid pronation and supination movements
- At 8 weeks weight bearing is allowed according to radiographic signs of ongoing fusion. The patient is gradually weaned off crutches. If a noncompleted fusion is seen on radiographs at this stage, a CAM boot can be used for a further 2–3 weeks
- Physical therapy is used for lower extremity rehabilitation
- At 3 months postoperatively final clinical and radiographic evaluations are carried out

Implant removal

- Hardware removal is rarely necessary

Myserson MS (ed.). Reconstructive foot and ankle surgery: management of complications, 2nd edn. Philadelphia: Elsevier Saunders, 2010.

Endoscopic and open calcaneoplasty

Indications

- Haglund's disease, which is defined as a clinical situation of tenderness and pain of the posterolateral calcaneus, involving a superolateral calcaneal prominence, retrocalcaneal bursitis, and an insertional tendinopathy of the Achilles tendon (van Dijk et al, 2001)
- Recalcitrant retrocalcaneal bursitis with an enlarged posterosuperior border of the os calcis without pain at the Achilles insertion

Contraindications

- Infection
- Open wounds or blisters
- Peripheral vascular disease

Preoperative assessment

Clinical assessment

Clinical presentation

- The patient usually complains of pain after walking, especially after a period of rest. The symptoms may worsen when walking up inclines
- The pain is localized slightly proximal to the insertion of the Achilles tendon on the calcaneus and is exacerbated when the patient performs a push-off or a single-legged heel raise
- Pain may also be reported at the retrocalcaneal bursa. Dorsiflexion of the foot causes the anterior part of the Achilles tendon to impinge on the posterosuperior rim of the calcaneus, thus producing a retrocalcaneal bursitis
- Pain may be evoked when the patient wears shoes
- A distinction between Haglund's syndrome and other pathologies of the posterolateral aspect of the heel must be made
- The differential diagnosis of posterior heel pain includes Achilles tendonitis, calcified Achilles tendon insertion, paratendonitis, conditions associated with seronegative spondyloarthritis such as Reiter's syndrome, psoriasic arthritis and ankylosing spondylitis (Siciliano, 1993)

Physical examination

- A preliminary observation of the patient's gait and characteristics is fundamental. You may observe a prominence on the heel, a callus, or erythema over the prominence caused by shoe wear
- The clinician should palpate the whole heel, foot, and Achilles tendon insertion, to identify tenderness, swelling, and nodularity
- A bony prominence may be palpable at the posterosuperior part of the calcaneus
- The Achilles tendon may become thicker, with loss of the clear interface with the adipose tissue
- When assessing the range of motion, the affected side is commonly seen to lose 5° of dorsiflexion compared to the normal side
- Hindfoot varus may predispose to the development of heel pain. Indeed, the calcaneus presents a marked vertical alignment in the cavus foot, causing a more prominent posterior projection (van Sterkenburg, 2012)

Imaging assessment

Radiographs

- Anteroposterior, lateral, and mortise ankle views and anteroposterior, lateral, and oblique weight-bearing views of the foot are required to show postero superior calcaneal prominence
- Possible calcifications at the Achilles tendon insertion or prominent posterior calcaneal tuberosity can be better assessed on the lateral views (**Figure 11.1**)
- Several radiographic angles and lines are used in evaluating the posterior calcaneus: for example, a Fowler–Philip's angle >75°, when the normal range is 44°–69°, a positive parallel

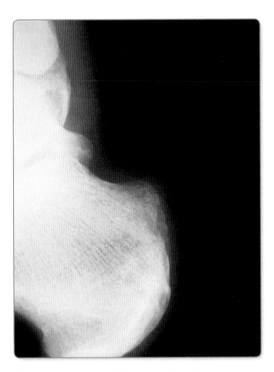

Figure 11.1 Evidence of Haglund's deformity.

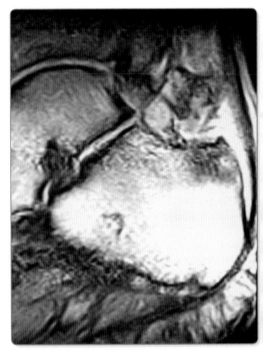

Figure 11.2 MRI: posterosuperior prominence of the calcaneus with bursitis.

pitch line, which is an osseous projection above the upper pitch line, or the calcaneal inclination angle. Nevertheless there is no consensus about the usefulness of these radiographic measurements

Magnetic resonance imaging (MRI)
- The loss of the retrocalcaneal recess may be evident on MRI and the normal signal intensity in the pre-Achilles fat pad area may be replaced by a soft tissue density
- Prominence of the posterosuperior calcaneus may also be identified (**Figure 11.2**)

Ultrasonography
- Ultrasonography may be useful for determining the status of the Achilles tendon, the retrocalcaneal bursa, and the cortex of the posterior aspect of the calcaneus

Timing for surgery
- It is used for recalcitrant cases that fail to improve after at least 6 months of conservative treatment
- The ankle range of motion must be normal

Surgical preparation
Special surgical considerations
- The first surgical technique for managing this condition was the *open* technique: an open resection calcaneoplasty of the dorsolateral side of the calcaneus, up to the Achilles tendon insertion. The *endoscopic* technique was subsequently developed in order to reduce invasiveness and postoperative morbidity
- The endoscopic technique is not recommended in the presence of calcific insertional Achilles tendinopathy, a partial or full rupture of the Achilles tendon, a posterior heel pain caused by rheumatologic pathologies, a cavus foot, or a varus foot

Surgical equipment
Open surgery equipment
- Needle holder
- Sutures
- Scalpels, blades no. 11 and 21

- Forceps: toothed tissue forceps, Adson's tissue forceps, Kocher's, Kelly's, and mosquito forceps
- Scissors
- Luer bone rongeur
- Farabeuf retractors
- Mini Hohmann bone elevators
- Bone curettes

Arthroscopic equipment

- Arthroscope
- Light source and cables
- Camera system and monitor
- Arthroscopic probe (hook)
- Arthroscopic punches (basket forceps)
- Arthroscopic grasper
- Motorized shaver
- Radio frequencies
- Arthroscopic burr

Equipment positioning

- The arthroscopic tower is positioned on the opposite side of the ankle, at the level of patient's contralateral hip
- The open surgery equipment is positioned near the surgeon, on the same side of the ankle to be operated on

Patient positioning

- The patient is placed in the prone position for both open surgery and endoscopic procedures
- The contralateral leg is abducted, so as not to interfere with the operative field
- The feet are positioned just at the edge of the operating table, in order to guarantee a neutral position of the ankle during the procedure
- A tourniquet is positioned on the proximal lower thigh

Further preparation

- The patient receives a single dose of intravenous antibiotics preoperatively
- Local or peripheral anesthesia is performed

Surgical technique

Open minimally invasive calcaneoplasty

- Local anesthestic is subcutaneously injected medially and laterally to the Achilles tendon (**Figure 11.3**)
- The thigh tourniquet is inflated

- Lateral longitudinal skin incision is made halfway between the proximal and the distal aspect of the calcaneus, extending proximally to the distal portion of the Achilles tendon
- After exposing the retrocalcaneal bursa (**Figure 11.4**), all soft tissues are removed from the bursal surface of the calcaneus until the tuberosity is visible
- A calcaneal osteotomy is then undertaken with a chisel, according to the preoperative planning (**Figure 11.5**)
- All sharp edges medially, laterally, and posteriorly are rounded off with a curette
- The surgeon should pay attention to the Achilles tendon insertion, verifying its anatomic integrity (**Figure 11.6**)

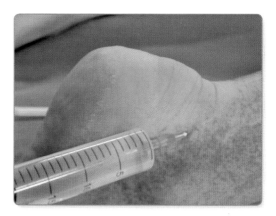

Figure 11.3 Local anesthesia.

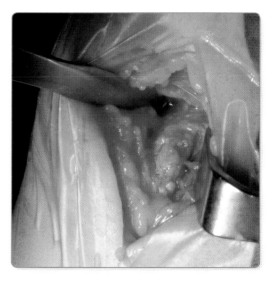

Figure 11.4 Exposition of the posterosuperior calcaneus.

- Fluoroscopy may be used to check the final result after calcaneoplasty (**Figure 11.7**)
- Debridement of fibrotic tissue should be performed cautiously
- Maximal dorsiflexion of the ankle should be performed intraoperatively to ensure that the osteotomy surface does not impinge on the Achilles tendon

- The wound is then irrigated and closed, without any drainage
- A well-padded, short leg cast is applied with the foot in the relaxed equinus position

Endoscopic calcaneoplasty

- Local anesthesia is used
- No tourniquet is necessary

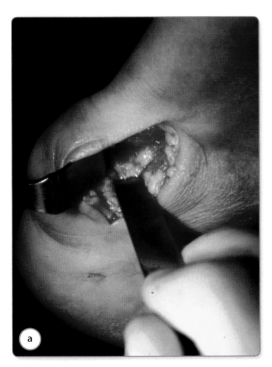

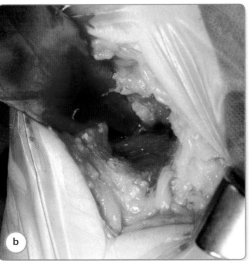

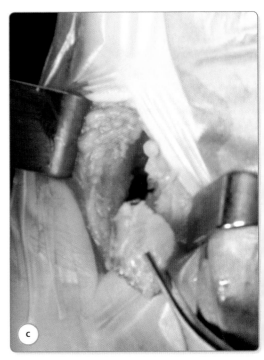

Figure 11.5 Calcaneal osteotomy. (a) Osteotomy with a chisel. (b) Calcaneus after the posterosuperior resection. The Achilles tendon insertional area is preserved. (c) The bone is excised.

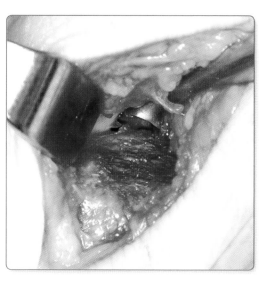

Figure 11.6 Curettage of the calcaneal margins; the Achilles tendon is carefully left untouched.

- Medial and lateral portals are set at the superior border of the calcaneal tuberosity on both sides of the Achilles tendon insertion
- The lateral portal is created through a small, vertical skin incision
- Using a blunt trocar, enter the retrocalcaneal space, irrigating it with a gravity flow or a pressured flow
- Under direct vision, a spinal needle is introduced medial to the Achilles tendon, establishing the medial portal (**Figure 11.8**)
- The optical camera is introduced through the portals
- The inflamed retorcalcaneal bursa is removed using basket forceps, which allows visualization of the superior aspect of the calcaneus
- A thorough synovectomy and a resection of the fibrous layer and periosteum are performed using a bone-cutter shaver, allowing a good visualization of the calcaneal prominence and the Achilles tendon
- The posterosuperior calcaneal rim is then removed with a barrel burr, without damaging the Achilles tendon insertion (**Figure 11.9**)
- It is important not to leave any sharp bony prominence on either side of the bone
- Excision adequacy is confirmed by the absence of impingement when the ankle is fully dorsiflexed

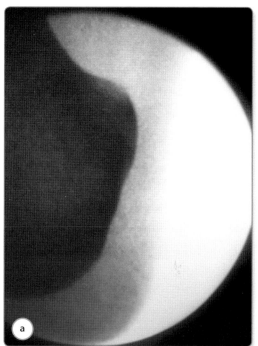

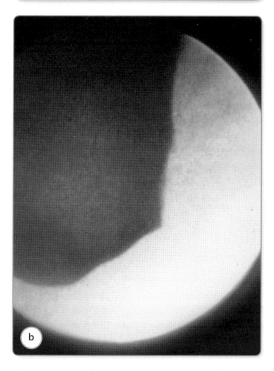

Figure 11.7 Radiologic evaluation before (a) and after (b) calcaneal osteotomy.

- The skin incisions are sutured and Steri-Strips are applied
- An elastic bandage is applied with the ankle in a neutral position (**Figure 11.10**)

Possible perioperative complications

- In comparison with the open procedure, endoscopic calcaneoplasty offers the advantages of low morbidity, excellent scar healing but no shorter recovery time, and quicker return to sport

- While performing the miniopen technique it is important not to damage the neurovascular structures
- There is a relative risk of damaging the sural nerve, which may be identified posterolaterally and protected (Morag, 2003)

Open mininvasive calcaneoplasty

- Skin breakdown
- Wound-healing problems, due to the poor blood supply to the posterior ankle area
- Retrocalcaneal bursitis
- Painful scar with sural neuritis

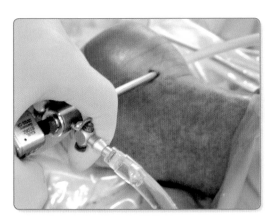

Figure 11.8 A trocar is inserted in to the retrocalcaneal space, slightly above the posterosuperior calcaneal margin.

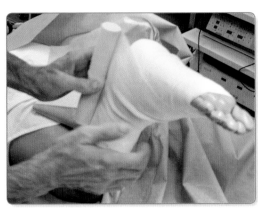

Figure 11.10 Elastic bandage applied after surgery.

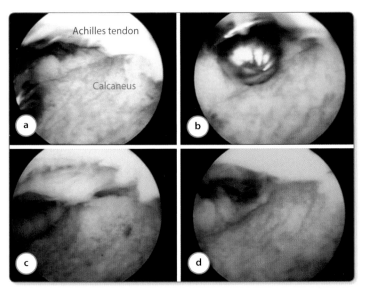

Figure 11.9 Sequence of surgery. (a) Retrocalcaneal space. (b) Calcaneoplasty with burr. (c) The calcaneus osseous prominence is progressively resected. (d) The insertional area is carefully preserved.

- Stiffness
- Achilles tendon avulsion
- Calcaneal (stress) fractures

Closure

- After thorough irrigation with normal saline, the skin incisions are sutured and Steri-Strips are applied
- A drain is not necessary. If the surgeon chooses to use it, a suction drain is not recommended as it can precipitate significant bleeding from the cancellous bone of the calcaneus (Jerosh, 2007)
- A pneumatic ankle brace or a light cast is applied
- An elastic bandage is always applied on the skin to avoid distal edema

Postoperative management

- Patient can immediately start partial weight bearing and begin ankle range of motion exercises as tolerated with full weight bearing in the 3rd week

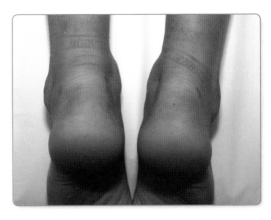

Figure 11.11 Bilateral case in a long-distance runner.

- Normal activities may be resumed at 4–6 weeks postoperatively
- Sport activities are usually resumed 2–4 months postoperatively (**Figure 11.11**)

Outpatient follow-up

- Patients are assessed at 6-month intervals for 2 years and can be discharged at that stage
- Further examinations will be necessary only if symptoms recur or if there is new trauma

Further reading

Jerosch J, Schunck J, Sokkar SH. Endoscopic calcaneoplasty (ECP) as a surgical treatment of Haglund's syndrome. Knee Surg Sports Traumatol Arthrosc. 2007; 15:927–934.

Morag G, Maman E, Arbel R. Endoscopic Treatment of Hindfoot Pathology. Arthroscopy. 2003;19(2):E13. Sella EJ, Caminear DS, McLarney EA. Haglund's syndrome. J Foot Ankle Surg 1998; 37:110–114.

Siciliano CJ, Mozen NA. Rheumatoid-like nodules presenting as Haglund's deformity in an adult, nonarthritic patient. J Foot Ankle Surg 1993; 32:484–489.

van Dijk CN, van Dijk GE, Scholten PE, et al. Endoscopic calcaneoplasty. Am J Sports Med 2001; 29:185–189.

van Sterkenburg MN, de Leeuw PAJ, van Dijk CN. Endoscopic Calcaneoplasty. In: Achilles tendinopathy: new insights in cause of pain, diagnosis and management, 2012.

Wu Z, Hua Y, Li Y, et al. Endoscopic treatment of Haglund's syndrome with a three portal technique. Int Orthop 2012; 36:1623–1627.

Indications

Os trigonum syndrome is characterized by pain, swelling, and tenderness to palpation at the posterior aspect of the ankle joint, just anterior to the Achilles tendon. Posterior endoscopic excision of a symptomatic os trigonum is indicated when:

- It causes a painful limitation of plantarflexion of the ankle

Preoperative assessment

Clinical assessment

- Physical examination reveals pain on palpation of the posterior aspect of the ankle just anterior to the Achilles tendon on both sides
- Plantar flexion range of movement may be reduced compared with contralateral joint
- The hyper plantar flexion test: repetitive, quick, and forced plantarflexion movements of the ankle with the knee flexed to 30°: it is considered positive if it evokes pain in maximum plantarflexion
- Differential diagnosis: Achilles tendonitis, retrocalcaneal bursitis, flexor hallucis longus (FHL) tenosynovitis, Haglund's disease, posterior tibial tendonitis, osteochondal lesions of the posterior talar dome, tarsal tunnel syndrome, tarsal coalition, and talus fracture
- The presence of considerable swelling on the medial aspect of the ankle just posterior to the medial malleolus is often related to an FHL tendon tenosynovitis or tear
- A fluoroscopically guided injection with 2 mL of lidocaine around the os trigonum is sometimes advocated to confirm the diagnosis. The diagnostic block is considered positive if patient experiences a temporary but significant relief of symptoms throughout the full range of motion

Imaging assessment

Radiographs

- Plain lateral radiographs of the ankle usually demonstrate the presence of an os trigonum
- Impingement of the os trigonum between the calcaneus and the posterior aspect of the tibia can be demonstrated with a lateral ankle radiograph with the ankle in forced plantarflexion (**Figure 12.1**)

Computed tomography (CT)

- CT can identify the extent of osseus involvement and help to distinguish between a true os trigonum and a fracture

Magnetic resonance imaging (MRI)

- MRI may be helpful to diagnose any associated injury such as FHL tenosynovitis, peroneal tendon tears, or soft tissue edema

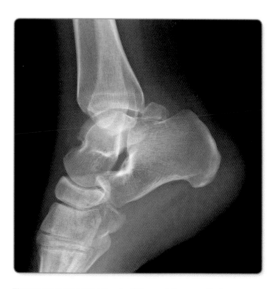

Figure 12.1 Impingement of the os trigonum between the calcaneus and the posterior aspect of the tibia can be proven with a radiograph in lateral view taken with the ankle in forced plantarflexion.

Timing for surgery

- Os trigonum syndrome is always treated conservatively at first
- Patients who are in pain and have failed conservative treatment for at least 6 months should be considered for surgical excision of the os trigonum

Surgical preparation

Surgical equipment

- A 4.0 mm or 2.7 mm 30° arthroscopic set is used
- In addition, a 4.0 mm dissector and 4.0 mm burr shaver blade are employed
- An arrthroscopic pump is not required. Adequate flow is obtained with gravity alone
- An ankle distractor is not routinely used

Equipment positioning

- The arthroscopic tower can be placed approximately at the level of the patient's shoulder at either side of the bed as the surgeon is usually at the distal end of the bed

Patient positioning

- The patient is placed in a prone position with the knee slightly flexed and the ankle over the distal end of the bed so that the ankle can be moved both in dorsal and plantarflexion (**Figure 12.2**)
- Care must be taken to ensure that the foot is perfectly perpendicular to the ground (**Figure 12.3**)

Further preparation

- Antibiotic prophylaxis is not routinely administered

Surgical technique

Portal placement

- The two posterior portals are located at the level of the tip of the medial and lateral malleolus as close as possible to the Achilles tendon on both sides (**Figure 12.4**)
- The posterolateral portal is the main viewing portal and is prepared first
- The posterolateral portal level should be checked under fluoroscopy (**Figure 12.5**) to allow not only the excision of the os trigonum

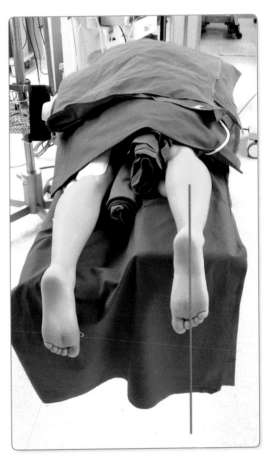

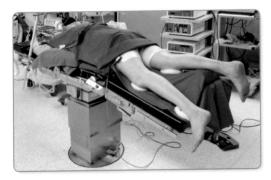

Figure 12.2 The ankle is placed over the distal end of the table with a small support under the leg.

Figure 12.3 The foot must be perpendicular to the ground.

but also ankle and posterior subtalar joint arthroscopy if needed. With some experience this step can be skipped

- A longitudinal incision is made, taking care to only cut the skin and avoid the Achilles tendon
- A blunt clamp is pushed forward, pointing to the posterolateral aspect of the ankle. When the tip of the clamp hits the bone it can be moved medially and laterally following the profile of the bone, to clear away the subcutaneous tissues
- The clamp is then removed and replaced with the arthroscope, again pointing to the posterolateral aspect of the ankle
- The posteromedial portal is made under direct vision with insertion of a needle to guide the direction and level of the skin incision. The level is usually the same as the posterolateral portal. The clamp is pushed onward around the anterolateral profile of the Achilles tendon until it touches the arthroscopic cannula. The clamp is then pushed anteriorly following the arthroscope until it contacts the bone surface
- The clamp is again removed and replaced with the shaver blade
- When an instrument is inserted through the posteromedial portal it should first touch the arthroscopic cannula just anteriorly to the Achilles tendon
- Follow the arthroscopic cannula until the instrument comes into view or os visible through the arthroscope

Preparation of the os trigonum

- With a 4.0 mm dissector shaver facing the bone, the fatty tissue is carefully removed. The crural fascia is then identified and opened just lateral to the posterior talar process enough to introduce the arthroscope and the shaver
- The posterolateral aspect of the os trigonum and the subtalar joint can be visualized. Eversion–inversion movements of the calcaneus can help identifying the subtalar joint (**Figure 12.6**)
- The posterior ankle joint is still not visible at this time as it is covered by the intermalleolar ligament and the transverse ligament. Elevating the two ligaments with a probe, the posterior ankle joint can be inspected. Forced

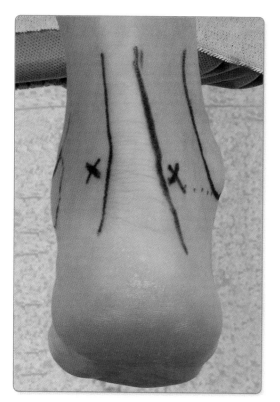

Figure 12.4 Portal placement.

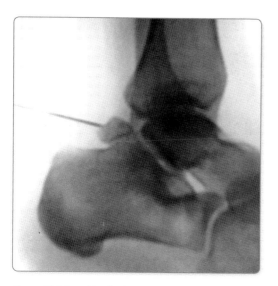

Figure 12.5 Portal levels checked under fluoroscopy.

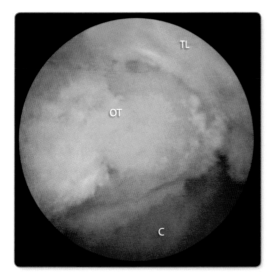

Figure 12.6 Posterolateral aspect of the os trigonum (OT) and subtalar joint. C, calcaneus; TL, transverse ligament.

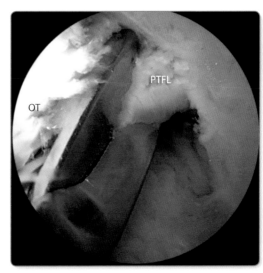

Figure 12.8 The posterior talofibular ligament (PTFL) is cut with a basket forceps. OT, os trigonum.

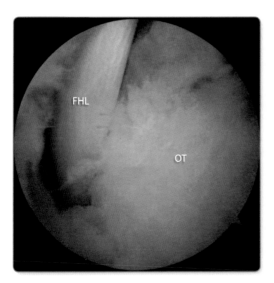

Figure 12.7 The flexor hallucis longus (FHL) tendon is identified just medial to the os trigonum (OT).

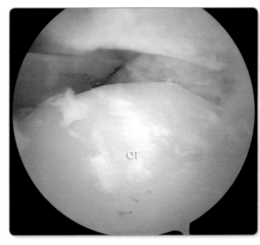

Figure 12.9 A small blunt osteotome can be used to release the synchondrosis between the posterior aspect of the talus and the os trigonum (OT).

dorsal flexion of the ankle allows visualization of the posterior half of the talar dome
- The soft tissues are removed by moving the shaver medially always following the bone profile until the FHL is identified. When moving the shaver medially, care must be taken not to pass the FHL tendon as just medial to it is the neurovascular bundle.

Flexion–extension of the great toe can help to identify the tendon. The area lateral to the FHL is a safe working area (**Figure 12.7**)

Os trigonum removal

- The os trigonum is released completely from its attachment to the posterior talo-fibular ligament, the flexor retinaculum, and the

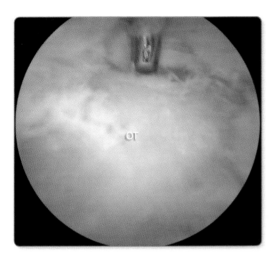

Figure 12.10 A probe is used to identify the synchondrosis. OT, os trigonum.

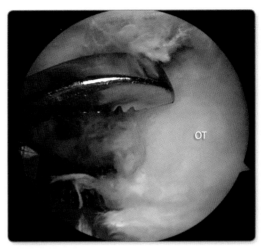

Figure 12.11 The os trigonum (OT) is removed with a grasper.

posterior talocalcanear ligament (**Figure 12.8**)
- Removal of the os trigonum also requires detachment from the posterior aspect of the talus with a small blunt osteotome (**Figure 12.9**). The fibrous fusion between the os trigonum and the posterior talus, if not visible, can be identified with a probe (**Figure 12.10**)
- The os trigonum is now completely mobile and it can be removed with a grasper (**Figure 12.11**)
- In cases where the os trigonum cannot be completely mobilized (or a Stieda's process is present) it can be removed with an arthroscopic burr and complete excision can be checked with fluoroscopy

Associated pathologies
- After excision of the os trigonum the posterior ankle joint and posterior subtalar joint can be inspected and any associated pathology (i.e. osteochondral lesion, loose bodies, synovitis) can be treated if necessary (**Figure 12.12**)
- The FHL tendon can be inspected by releasing the flexor retinaculum and the tendon sheath. The proximal part of the tendon from the muscle belly to the groove can be inspected and debrided if needed (**Figure 12.13**)

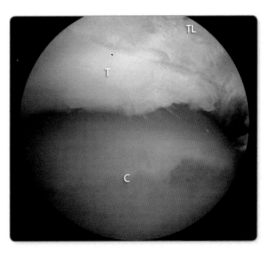

Figure 12.12 Inspection of posterior subtalar joint. C, calcaneus; T, talus; TL, transverse ligament.

Possible perioperative complications
- FHL tendon and peroneal tendon injury: Debride and suture if possible; otherwise convert to an open procedure
- Neurovascular bundle injury: Convert to an open procedure and repair

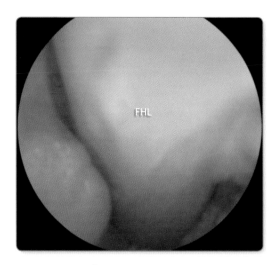

Figure 12.13 The flexor hallucis longus (FHL) tendon in its groove.

Closure

- Drainage is not needed
- Suture with 3-0 nylon
- An elastic compression bandage is applied from above the metatarsophalangeal joint

to below the knee, including the head of the fibula and taking care to carefully pad the perimalleolar region. Compression must decrease in pressure from distal to proximal and not constrict the leg

Postoperative management

- Medication: analgesia for 2–3 days if necessary (i.e. tramadol 50 mg every 6 hours), deep vein thrombosis prophylaxis with enoxaparin sodium for 15 days
- Active movement of the ankle from the first day after surgery
- Nonweight bearing

Outpatient follow-up

- 2 weeks: suture removal; weight-bearing as tolerated; full range of motion; closed-chain exercises such as cyling and swimming
- 4 weeks: running
- 6 weeks: sport-specific training
- 8 weeks: return to full sports activity

Further reading

Lundeen RO. Arthroscopic excision of the os trigonum. In: Guhl JF, Parisien JS, Boynton MD (eds), Foot and ankle arthroscopy. New York: Springer, 2004:191–199.

Sitler DF, Amendola A, Bailey CS, et al. Posterior ankle arthroscopy: an anatomic study. J Bone Joint Surg Am 2002; 84A:763–769.

van Dijk CN, Scholten PE, Krips R. A 2-portal endoscopic approach for diagnosis and treatment of posterior ankle pathology. Arthroscopy 2000; 16:871–876.

| | | | |

13 Accessory navicular bone excision

Indications

The accessory navicular bone is an accessory nucleus of ossification with interposed fibroconnective tissue and occasionally cartilage, located on the medial side of the foot. It is continuous with the tibialis posterior tendon (**Figure 13.1**).

It is also associated with cavus valgus foot and unilateral pes planus and may become symptomatic due to mechanical pressure against footwear. Pain can also be caused by degenerative tendinopathy of tibialis posterior (**Figure 13.2**).

Symptoms of accessory navicular bone may also be exacerbated by trauma. Simultaneous eversion and tibialis posterior tendon contraction can fracture the attachment of the ossicle, causing a diastasis of the accessory navicular resulting in abnormal motion and pain (**Figure 13.3**).

The indications for surgical excision are:

- Symptomatic accessory navicular bone due to rubbing on footwear
- In combination with the correction of flat foot
- Secondary medial tarsalgia due to tibialis posterior tendinopathy

Preoperative assessment

Clinical assessment

- The patient presents with medial tarsalgia, which is accentuated by walking
- Physical examination shows a pronated foot when walking
- Pain is elicited on palpation of the medial navicular tubercle

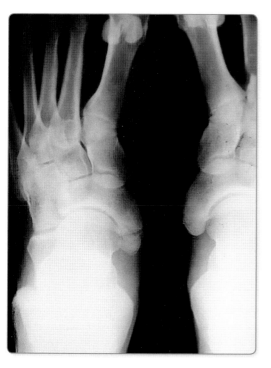

Figure 13.1 Dorsoplantar radiographs show the presence of an accessory navicular in the left foot, and its assimilation in right foot.

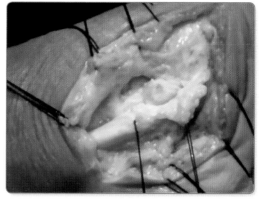

Figure 13.2 An image of degenerative glenophaty on a microtraumatic basis.

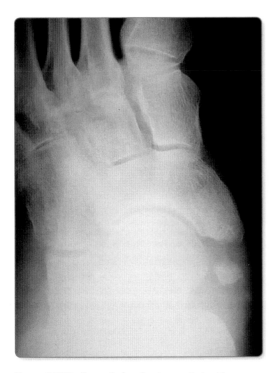

Figure 13.3 Radiograph showing traumatic traction.

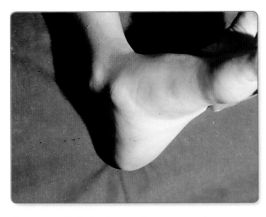

Figure 13.4 Clinical evidence of an accessory bone.

A bony swelling is often visible on the medial aspect of the navicular, with associated erythema (**Figure 13.4**).

Imaging assessment

- Weight-bearing dorsoplantar and lateral radiographs of the foot are sufficient to identify an accessory navicular bone

- The radiographs may demonstrate a hypertrophied medial navicular ossification center as well as its size and position
- Radiographs may not be useful if the accessory navicular is not ossified
- CT and MRI are indicated if there is suspicion of other foot pathologies (**Figure 13.1**)
- A bone scan may be useful if it is unclear whether an accessory navicular is causing symptoms

Timing for surgery

- Failure of non operative treatment such as orthotics is an indication
- A symptomatic accessory navicular bone which is painful and is rubbing on footwear should be treated
- Excision can be undertaken early in children especially if associated with cavus-valgus or a flexible pes planus

Surgical preparation

Surgical equipment

- Scalpel
- Dissecting scissors
- Klemmer's forceps
- Oscillating saw
- Sharp chisels
- Hammer
- Metal staples

Equipment positioning

- We prefer to place all surgical instruments required to perform surgery on a small serving table in front of the foot, for the operation

Patient positioning

- The patient is placed in the supine position
- A tourniquet is applied to the upper thigh

Surgical technique

Exposure

- The Kidner operation is used to remove the accessory navicular bone
- A curvilinear S-shaped incision is made which extends from below the medial malleolous to the medial cuneiform (**Figure 13.5**)
- The medial malleolus, the sheath, and the tendon of the tibialis posterior, the

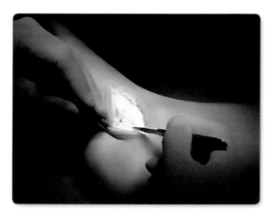

Figure 13.5 Surgical medial approach with a curvilinear S-shaped incision.

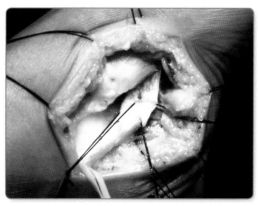

Figure 13.7 The operating field showing the navicular and glenoid.

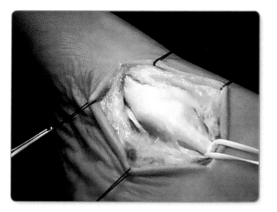

Figure 13.6 The exposed tibial posterior tendon and the tubercle of the scaphoid.

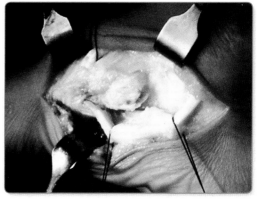

Figure 13.8 Exposure of the accessory navicular.

medial tubercle of the navicular, the medial cuneiform, and, lying plantar, the muscle belly of the hallux adductor covered by its fascia, are all exposed (**Figure 13.6**)
- Retraction of the skin is achieved by tethering the edges using silk sutures

Deep dissection
- The tibialis posterior sheath is then opened and is detached from the medial tubercle of the navicular without interrupting its continuity with the distal and lateral insertions
- The lateral expansion of the tibialis posterior tendon is sutured using silk, allowing for retraction. This allows visualization of the navicular, talus, and plantar calcanonavicular ligament (**Figure 13.7**)

Resection of the navicular
- The accessory navicular is exposed (**Figure 13.8**) and removed with a scalpel along the course of the fibrous coalescence
- Exposure of the accessory navicular bone can sometimes be difficult due it being located plantar to the medial tubercle of the navicular. In this case, a tangential sliver of the medial tubercle can be removed in order to locate the plane between the accessory navicular and the medial tubercle. Sometimes there are difficulties in exposing the accessory scaphoid bone because it is plantar to the medial tubercle of the scaphoid (**Figure 13.9**)
- In the presence of a large or plantar accessory navicular bone, complete excision may

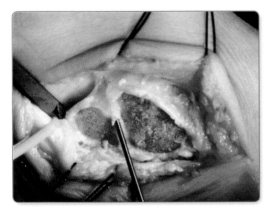

Figure 13.9 An accessory navicular plantar to the medial tubercle.

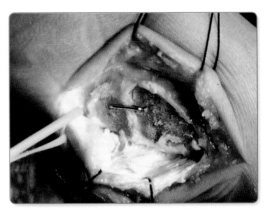

Figure 13.10 A highly voluminous accessory navicular and its arthrodesis with a staple.

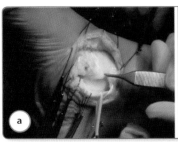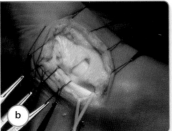

Figure 13.11 (a) Evaluation of capsule-ligament laxity. (b) Full-thickness orthogonal excision.

result in a further loss of stability of the coxa pedis with possible development into talar protrusion. In this case a simple tangential resection of the accessory navicular bone is performed and the bone is fused to the medial tubercle of the navicular with a metal staple (**Figure 13.10**)

- At this point, the capsule–ligament laxity is evaluated and affects the tibial–navicular component of the deltoid ligament (**Figure 13.11a**)
- A full-thickness orthogonal excision of the capsule is performed in a medial crescent shape, parallel to the scaphoid, to allow sufficient anchoring tissue for the subsequent tendon reconstruction (**Figure 13.11b**)

Possible perioperative complications

- The most frequent intraoperative complication is injury to the posterior tibial tendon during its detachment from the medial pole of the navicular
- There is potential destabilization of the midfoot after removal of a large accessory navicular bone

Closure

- The capsule is closed using interrupted vertical mattress sutures from proximal to distal with a slow-absorption suture material. Closure of the capsule under tension provides stability (**Figure 13.12a**)
- The tibialis posterior tendon is then sutured under tension to the capsule and previously exposed lateral expansion of tibialis posterior. Alternatively, the tendon can be attached to the bone using bone anchors (**Figure 13.12b**)
- The tibialis posterior tendon is then placed back into its tendinous sheath, which is then reconstructed
- The subcutaneous tissues are then closed using a absorbable suture, and the skin with

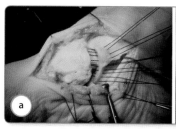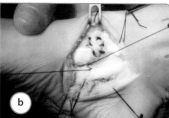

Figure 13.12 (a) Suture with U-shaped stitches. (b) Re-tensioning stitch on lateral branch of tibialis posterior.

an interrupted nonabsorbable monofilament, which is removed 2 weeks postoperatively

Postoperative management

- Immobilization is in a synthetic below-knee splint for 3 weeks. Nonweight bearing lasts for 6 weeks
- At 3 weeks the spint is removed and the patient is allowed to begin active and passive movement

- This is followed by progressively increasing weight bearing until full weight bearing is tolerated

Outpatient follow-up

- 2-week follow-up for wound review and removal of sutures
- 6-week follow-up at the beginning of weight bearing

Further reading

Pisani G. Trattato di chirurgia del piede, 3rd edn. Torino: Edizioni Minerva Medica, 2004.

Pisani G, Pisani PC, Parino E. Degenerative pathology of the "coxa pedis". A new pathological entity. Eur Musculoskelet Rev 2008; 3:71–73.

Tryfonidis M, Jackson W, Mansour R, et al. Acquired adult flat foot due to isolate plantar calcaneo-navicular (spring) ligament insufficiency with a normal tibialis posterior tendon. Foot Ankle Surg 2006; 14:89–95.

Open plantar excision of Morton's neuroma

Indications

- Morton's symptoms – defined as pain in the intermetatarsal space and in the adjacent toes while walking
- Failure of at least 6 months of conservative management, including steroid injections, shoe adaptations, and orthoses
- It is important to consider other, neurologic causes which may eventually result in forefoot pain, i.e. lumbar radiculopathy or tarsal tunnel syndrome (Amis, 1994)

Risk factors

- Nerve compression secondary to swelling of the intermetatarsal bursa (Betts, 1940)
- Vascular injuries (Nissen, 1948)
- More common in women, with an onset of symptoms in the fifth decade

Contraindications

- There may be symptomatic overlap between Morton's symptoms and other forefoot pathology that causes increased pressure under the metatarsal heads, e.g. hyperplantar keratosis, metatarsalgia, synovitis, or metatarsophalangeal joint bursitis
- Pathologies may coexist but require different treatments
- Any extrinsic inflammation or compression of an interdigital nerve may cause nerve irritation, leading to clinical signs which are similar to those of an interdigital neuroma

Preoperative assessment

Clinical assessment

Clinical presentation

- Symptoms include:
  - A burning, aching or cramping pain occurs between a pair of metatarsal heads, most commonly the third web space
  - The classical description is that it is like walking with a stone in the shoe
  - The pain is often relieved by resting and removing the shoes
  - An intermittent paresthesia usually affects the third web space
- The duration of symptoms ranges from a few weeks to many years

Physical examination

- A comparative evaluation of both feet should be performed, including the hind - mid - and forefoot
- In particular, the clinician should inspect for deviation or subluxation of the toes or fullness of the web space
- The most common physical finding is plantar tenderness on direct palpation or on stretching the toes around the affected web space
- A useful maneuver to distinguish a metatarsophalangeal joint synovitis from a neuroma requires plantarflexion of the relevant joint: if synovitis is present, this movement causes a burning pain, while in the presence of a neuroma the pain rises gradually
- Mulder's test or Mulder's click – squeezing across the foot at the level of the metatarsal heads may elicit a palpable click
- The Tinel–Hoffmann sign evokes a sensation of 'pins and needles' over the nerve trunk after tapping over the suspected web space
- Very few cases of metatarsal pain are caused by Morton's neuroma (Canata and Ciclamini, 2005)

Imaging assessment

- There is some debate as to the best imaging method, but the most commonly mentioned are ultrasonography and MRI
- Some research suggests that ultrasonography and MRI are specific and sensitive enough for a correct Morton's neuroma diagnosis
- Recently, several studies have reported a large variation in the sensitivity and specificity

of MRI and ultrasonography; thus the best diagnostic imaging technique is still debatable
- Because of the low correlation between these two tests, some authors suggest that MRI and ultrasonography might enhance each other. Thus the technique of choice for an accurate diagnosis is to perform both (Torres-Claramunt et al, 2012)
- Other tests include computerized tomography CT injection of local anesthetics, and electrophysiologic tests, i.e electromyography (Torres-Claramunt et al, 2012)

Ultrasonography

- Radiologic investigations are particularly useful when pain is perceived at several web spaces or if the clinical history is equivocal
- Ultrasonography is less expensive and allows real-time localization of the neuroma
- On the other hand, ultrasonography is a 'user-dependent' test, so it has been suggested that it may lead to an overestimation of the neuroma's size (Read, 1999)
- Sonographic parameters for Morton's neuroma are:
  - A focal hypoechoic nodule replacing the hyperechoic interdigital fat of the web space of the forefoot at the metatarsal heads (Torres-Claramunt et al, 2012)
  - Inflammatory fibrosis surrounding the interdigital nerve by the distal extension of the transverse intermetatarsal ligament
  - Heterogenous echogenicity

Magnetic resonance imaging (MRI)

- The most common findings are contrast enhancement and abnormal signal intensity of the structures in the web space affected (**Figure 14.1**)
- The best visibility of a Morton's neuroma is obtained with the patient placed in the prone position

Radiographs

- Because of the nature of the involved structures, radiographs are not usually indicated; nevertheless they may be employed to rule out possible bony pathology
- The standard radiologic examinations are the anteroposterior, lateral, and oblique projections

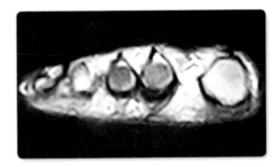

Figure 14.1 MRI with evidence of a neuromatous formation in the third intermetatarsal web space.

Computed tomography (CT)

- CT may be helpful only if there are residual diagnostic doubts. A deep scan may exclude suspected bony processes, such as an early Freiberg's infraction (Amis, 1994)

Timing for surgery

- Surgery takes place only if the conservative treatment has failed
- The re should be integrity of the other anatomic structures

Surgical preparation

Special surgical considerations

- The first step is choosing between the dorsal and the plantar approach
- The former has the advantage of low wound complications, a lower incidence of plantar scar formation, and immediate weight bearing after the surgical treatment
- The latter is more direct, less dissection is required, and it preserves the transverse metatarsal ligament, thus ensuring a lower incidence of instability (Jackson, 2013)
- Whichever approach is used, a tissue release with decompression can be combined with a metatarsal shortening osteotomy and a neurectomy
- After neurectomy, the removed material is sent to the laboratory to check its histologic nature and to confirm the diagnosis

Surgical equipment

- Needle holder

- Sutures
- Scalpel, blades no. 11 and 21
- Forceps: toothed tissue forceps, Adson's tissue forceps, Kocher's, Kelly's, and mosquito forceps
- Scissors
- Farabeuf retractors
- Mini Hohmann bone elevators

Equipment positioning

- The surgical equipment is positioned near the surgeon, at the same side of the ankle to be operated on

Patient positioning

- The patient is placed in the supine position
- A tourniquet is positioned on the thigh
- At the appropriate time, the foot, ankle, and leg are exsanguinated and the tourniquet is inflated

Further preparation

- The patient receives a single dose of intravenous antibiotics preoperatively
- Local anesthesia can be infiltrated pre- or postoperatively

Surgical technique

Tissue dissection

- A 3–4 cm longitudinal plantar incision is made over the affected intermetatarsal space, on the distal fat pad and far from the weight-bearing area (**Figure 14.2**)
- The dissection is deepened with scissors until the fibers of the superficial transverse intermetatarsal ligaments are identified (Boberg, 1995)
- After dissecting the fibers, the interspace is assessed to identify the vessels and the common digital nerve with its proper digital branches
- The common digital nerve lies in a plantar position to the intermetatarsal ligament, superficial to the flexor digitorum brevis muscle and deep to the plantar fascia

Neurectomy

- The neuroma is identified and dissected visualizing proximal and distal branches (**Figure 14.3**)
- The two distal branches of the nerve are sectioned and a clamp is applied

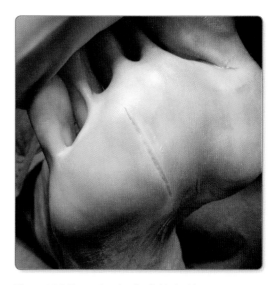

Figure 14.2 Plantar longitudinal skin incision.

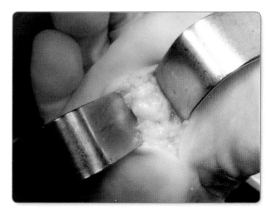

Figure 14.3 Visualization of the neuromatous formation after tissue dissection.

- The common digital nerve is distracted distally and the subcutaneous tissues are dissected proximally (**Figure 14.4**). The common digital nerve trunk is now sectioned proximal to the metatarsal heads
- It is important to transect the neuroma as close as possible to the nerve bifurcation (**Figure 14.5**)
- The ideal transecting distance is 3 cm proximal to the closest border of the intermetatarsal ligament
- This maneuver allows resection of the plantar branches to guarantee nerve stump retraction far from the weight-bearing area

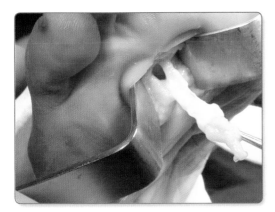

Figure 14.4 Proximal and distal section of the neuroma.

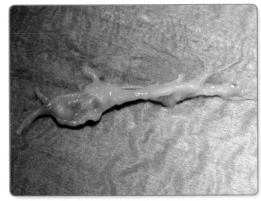

Figure 14.5 The removed Morton's neuroma.

- Generally, the resected neuroma is analyzed histologically to confirm the diagnosis

Possible perioperative complications

- Sectioning the deep transverse intermetatarsal ligament, as occurs through the dorsal approach, modifies the mechanical characteristics of the lumbrical tendon
- The incision site presents several anatomic structures to be preserved during surgery: the proper plantar digital branches of the medial or lateral nerve (depending on the Morton's neuroma location), the lumbrical tendons, and, more deeply, the transverse head of the adductor hallucis

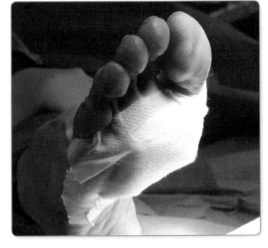

Figure 14.6 Postoperative medication before the elastic bandage application.

Closure

- The tourniquet is deflated and hemostasis is performed if necessary
- After thorough irrigation with 0.9% saline, the skin incision is sutured, Steri-Strips and medication are applied. Finally, an elastic bandage is wrapped (**Figure 14.6**)
- No buried sutures are used, in order to minimize the risk of fibrotic nodule formation in the subcutaneous tissues
- A compressive elastic bandage is always applied to avoid distal edema and development of a hematoma. The ankle is in the neutral position (**Figure 14.7**)

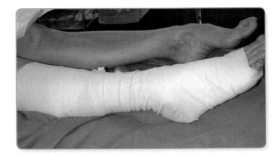

Figure 14.7 The postoperative elastic bandage: a cavus deformity is evident in both feet.

Postoperative management

Postoperative regimen

- Immediately after surgery the patient can be allowed to weightbear on the heel
- First 2 weeks postoperatively: Ice, elevation of the foot, medications such as pain relievers and nonsteroidal anti-inflammatory drugs thrombosis and pulmonary embolism prevention, and use of crutches are advised
- 2 weeks after surgery: Progressive forefoot weight bearing and removal of the sutures (**Figure 14.8**) are undertaken
- During rehabilitation, it is fundamental to begin early toe flexion and to avoid painful loads
- 1 month after surgery: A return to sport is allowed

Early-phase postoperative complications

- Wound breakdown
- Infection
- Bleeding
- Nerve injury
- Recurrence
- Complex regional pain syndrome

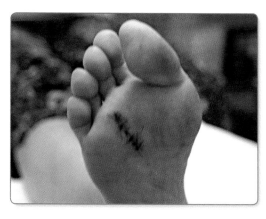

Figure 14.8 Skin incision after 2 week: the sutures are ready to be removed.

Outpatient follow-up

- Patients are assessed and discharged as seen fit – usually no more than 6-8 weeks of follow-up is required
- Further examinations will be necessary only if symptoms develop again or if a new trauma occurs

Further reading

Amis JA. Primary interdigital neuroma resection. In: Johnson KA (Ed.) Master techniques in orthopaedic surgery: the foot and ankle, 1st edn. Raven Press, New York 1994: 163–177.

Betts LO. Morton's metatarsalgia: neuritis of the 4th digital nerve. Med J Aust 1940; 1:514–515.

Boberg JS. Plantar Longitudinal Incision for Morton's Neuroma. Decatur: Podiatry Institute,1995. Philadelphia: Lippincott Williams & Wilkins, 2013.

Canata GL, Ciclamini D. Trattamento day surgery della syndrome di Morton in anestesia locale. In: La chirurgia mini-invasiva del piede e della caviglia. Bologna: Aulo Gaggi Editore 2005; 14:77–83.

Jackson L, Schaller TM. Surgery for Morton Neuroma Treatment & Management. New York: Medscape Orthopedics, 2013.

Nissen KI. Plantar digital neuritis; Morton's metatarsalgia. J Bone Joint Surg Br 1948; 30:84–94.

Read JW, Noakes JB, Kerr D, et al. Morton's metatarsalgia: sonographic findings and correlated histopathology. Foot Ankle Int 1999; 20:153–161.

Torres-Claramunt R, Ginés A, Pidemunt G, Puig L, de Zabala S. MRI and ultrasonography in Morton's neuroma: diagnostic accuracy and correlation. Indian J Orthop 2012; 46:321–325.

Indications

- Hallux valgus deformity according to the Italian Society of Orthopaedics and Traumatology guidelines
- Related conditions, i.e metatarsal overload, metatarsal pain, subluxation of one or more metatarsophalangeal (MTP) joints, and hammer toe

Surgical considerations

- The choice of the proper surgical treatment should be evaluated among:
  - Open surgery
  - Open minimally invasive surgery (MIS; i.e. simple, effective, rapid, inexpensive [SERI]/Bosch technique)
  - Closed MIS
- On the basis of the American Foot and Ankle Surgery and European Foot and Ankle Surgery guidelines the Spanish school suggests the evaluation of the following parameters:
  - Measurement of the hallus valgus angle (HVA): mild, HVA <20°, moderate, HVA >20° and <40°; severe, HVA >40°
  - Age of patient (younger or older than 50 years)
  - Type of sport or job activity
  - Symptoms
  - Radiologic anatomy of the foot

Preoperative assessment

Clinical assessment

- Hallux valgus with frequent dislocation of the sesamoids due to first toe pronation
- Hallux insufficiency with load transfer to the metatarsal bones associated with hammer toe
- Hyperkeratosis and medial bursitis caused by medial exostosis of the first metatarsal head
- The presence of hallux interphalangeus

Imaging assessment

Radiographs

- Anteroposterior, lateral, and oblique weight bearing radiographs of both feet. Values to evaluate:
  - Metatarsophalangeal angle or valgus angle (MTP angle/HVA): normal range <20°
  - Intermetatarsal angle (IMA or IMT): normal range <20° (**Figure 15.1**)
  - Proximal articular set angle (PASA): normal range <8° (**Figure 15.2**)
  - Distal articular set angle (DASA): normal range <8° (**Figure 15.3**)
  - Possible presence of exostosis
  - External dislocation of sesamoids

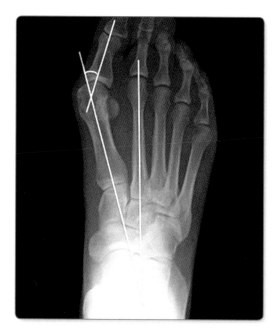

Figure 15.1 Anteroposterior standing radiographs: measurement of hallux valgus angle and first intermetatarsal angle.

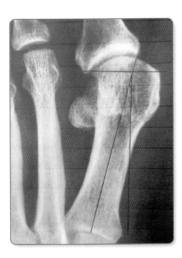

Figure 15.2
Lateral oblique radiograph: measurement of proximal articular set angle.

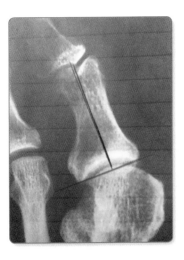

Figure 15.3
Lateral oblique radiograph: measurement of distal articular set angle.

- Congruence of the MTP joint (a positional deformity is present when the lines representing the articular surface of the first metatarsal head and the base of the proximal are not exactly parallel)

Timing for surgery

Choice of the surgical technique and timing is based on clinical and radiologic assessment.

- On patients younger than 50 years with HVA <20°, IMT <20°, and PASA >8°:
  - Bursectomy, exostosectomy, hallux abductor tenotomy, distal metaphyseal osteotomy of the first metatarsal (Reverdin–Isham technique). If the DASA is >8°, we will perform proximal metaphyseal

osteotomy of the proximal phalanx (Akin technique)
- With patients younger than 50 years with HVA 20–40°, IMT >20°, and PASA >8°:
  - Bursectomy, exostectomy, hallux abductor tenotomy, distal metaphyseal osteotomy of the first metatarsal (Reverdin–Isham technique), or proximal metaphyseal osteotomy of the first metatarsal. If the DASA is >8°, we will perform proximal metaphyseal osteotomy of the proximal phalanx (Akin technique)
- With patients older than 50 years with normal physical demands, HVA of any degree with IMT >20° (or >20° in a patient with poor physical demands), and PASA ≥8°:
  - Bursectomy, exostosectomy, distal metaphyseal osteotomy of the first metatarsal (Reverdin–Isham technique). If the DASA is >8° we will perform proximal metaphyseal osteotomy of the first phalange (P1) (Akin technique)
- With patients older than 50 years with high physical demands with an HVA 20–40°, IMT >20°, and PASA >8°:
  - Bursectomy, exostctomy, distal metaphyseal osteotomy of the first metatarsal (Reverdin–Isham technique), or proximal metaphyseal osteotomy of the first metatarsal. If the DASA is >8°, we will perform proximal metaphyseal osteotomy of the proximal phalanx (Akin technique)
- With patients older than 50 years with poor physical demands or comorbidity, with an HVA >40° and IMT >20°, in spite of the guidelines recommended by the Spanish school, the authors prefer the SERI or Bosch technique, which is a mini-invasive but open surgery

Surgical preparation

Surgical equipment

MIS surgical equipment

- Fluoroscopic X-ray machine
- Stimulator
- Beaver scalpel
- Wedge burr 4.1 × 13 mm
- Straight Shannon burr 2.0 × 12 mm
- Short Shannon burr 2.0 × 0.8 mm
- Long Shannon burr 2.0 × 12 mm

- Periosteal elevator (separator)
- Bone rasp 1.5 mm in width

SERI/Bosch surgical equipment
- Luer bone rongeur
- Farabeuf retractors
- Mini Hohmann bone elevators
- Hand drill
- Drill guide
- Kirschner (K)-wires
- Oscillating/reciprocating saw

Equipment positioning
- Fluoroscope positioning (MIS technique): in line with the operating table, distal to the patient, with the patient's foot lying on the fluoroscope support to allow plain radiographs

Patient positioning
- Patient positioning: the patient lies supine, with their feet slightly apart and lying off the edge of the operating table. The foot rests directly on the fluoroscope, which has had a sterile drape applied
- Anesthesia: perform sensory and motor block with 2 mg rovipacaine in 10 mL of injected solution at the level of the bifurcation of the sciatic nerve into the tibial nerve and common peroneal nerve, with the aid of a stimulator and an ultrasound system

Surgical technique: percutaneous minimally invasive technique (MIS)

- Disinfect accurately the foot skin including the interdigital spaces and prepare the surgical field
- Cover the X-ray unit with sterile drapes
- Place the tourniquet centrally around the leg, to be inflated only if necessary
- Under radiographic control, three 18G needles are positioned as radiologic and anatomic reference for the three main incisions (one medial below the head of the first metatarsal (MT), one lateral above the MTP joint, and one medial on the proximal metaphysis of the proximal phalanx) (**Figure 15.4**)
- Once the correct position of the needles has been identified under radiographic guidance, use a beaver scalpel to make the first 3 mm

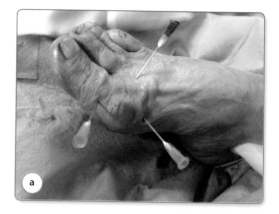

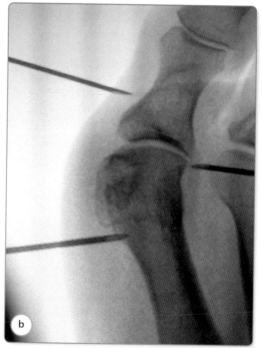

Figure 15.4 (a) Needles positioned before making any definitive incisions. (b) Radiographic control after needle positioning.

medial subcapital incision. This first incision is made from the base of the first metatarsal head running the blade distally (**Figure 15.5**)
- Introduce the separator following the same direction and detach both the subcutaneous bursal tissue and the capsular tissue of the MTP joint
- A wedge burr (4.1 mm) is inserted in to the space obtained. Milling between 1500 and

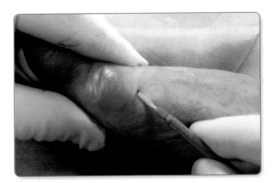

Figure 15.5 First incision medially to the metatarsophalangeal joint.

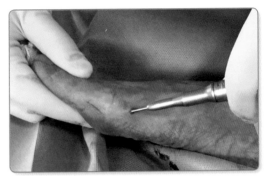

Figure 15.6 Exostosis drilling with the burr.

8000 rpm allows the removal of the tissue pouring from the access and the bone material corresponding to the exostosis. A deeper milling of the medial side of the metatarsal head may be useful to avoid bony painful protrusions at the joint level (**Figure 15.6**)

- Chiefly important is keeping the drill at intermediate speed to prevent damage to the skin caused by friction or overheating
- Through abundant and repeated washing as well as squeezing of the MTP region, debris, appearing as a bony and bloody paste, is removed
- Subsequently a second 3 mm incision is made laterally to the MTP joint of the hallux
- Insert a beaver scalpel, first with the blade parallel to the major axis of the proximal phalanx to perform a tenotomy of the adductor hallucis tendon, and then perform a large capsulotomy of the MTP joint, turning the blade 90° medially (**Figure 15.7**)
- Once the partial joint release is assessed, return to the initial incision
- Perform a periosteum dissection of the first MT neck with a specific rectum bone detacher (a soft tissue dissector)
- Using the straight Shannon burr (2.0 mm), a subcapital osteotomy of the first MT is performed from the medial to the lateral cortex, parallel to the PASA on the anteroposterior plane and at 45° oblique to the sagittal plane. The integrity of the lateral cortex should be carefully preserved (**Figure 15.8**)
- Holding the first metatarsal with both hands, complete the osteotomy manually, bringing

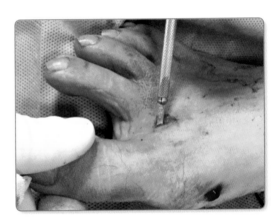

Figure 15.7 The second incision is performed on the lateral side of the first metatarsophalangeal joint.

the first ray in to varus. This maneuver creates a typical and perceptible sound when the cortex breaks. It allows the metatarsal to be realigned and centered over the sesamoids

- If the DASA is >8° and further correction of the valgus is required, an Akin osteotomy of the proximal phalanx is performed. Make a 3 mm medial access to the P1 proximal metaphysic with a beaver scalpel (**Figure 15.9**), dissect the tissues using the periosteal elevator and perform the osteotomy from the medial to the lateral cortex with a straight Shannon burr (2.0 mm). The lateral cortex is temporarily preserved (**Figure 15.10**)
- Complete the osteotomy manually to correct the DASA and slight varus alignment of the proximal phalanx

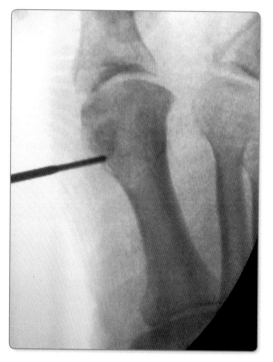

Figure 15.8 X-ray position checking of the straight Shannon burr.

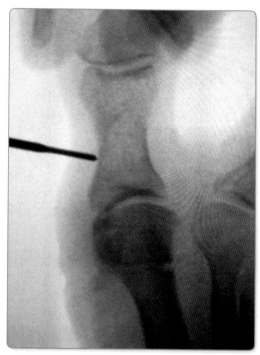

Figure 15.10 Radiographic control of the burr position before performing the osteotomy.

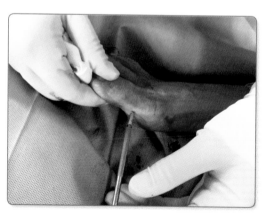

Figure 15.9 The third access at the P1 level to perform Akin osteotomy.

- If a wider correction is required (DASA >8° and HVA 20–40°), then perform a complete osteotomy in order to translate the whole proximal phalanx distal fragment

Closure

- Wash the surgical portals abundantly to remove any bone debris
- The small skin incisions do not require sutures
- Soft tissues infiltration with rovipacaine is performed around the osteotomy sites
- The foot is enclosed in a first layer of semi-circular bandage. A second layer of gauze is applied into the first and second interdigital spaces and tensioned medially, forcing the hallux in to varus without any plantar or dorsal deviation. The gauze must not be marked with lead wire or it will impede any radiographic images
- Soaking both the first and second layers of gauze with iodopovidone solution will harden the bandage after drying to keep the correction obtained (**Figure 15.11**)
- A circular elastic bandage and a further layer of gauze are applied into the first and the second interdigital spaces

- Final radiographic evaluation must be performed to ensure that the HVA has been corrected

Surgical technique: minimally invasive open technique (Bosch or SERI)

- Preparation and disinfection of the patient is exactly comparable to the previous one, except for the fluoroscopy machine, as the surgery is performed 'on sight'
- Inflate the tourniquet after squeezing the limb with an Esmarch bandage
- A 3 cm incision is centered over the medial side of the first MTP joint, exposing and removing the bursal tissue by blunt dissection
- Expose the neck of the first metatarsal bone using the periosteal elevator
- Perform a 2 cm incision in the first interdigital space and make a tenotomy of the adductor hallucis tendon

- A subcapital osteotomy of the first metatarsal is performed with a reciprocating or oscillating saw (**Figure 15.12**)
- After performing a medial dislocation of the distal fragment, insert a Kirschner (K)-wire (usually 1.6–1.8 mm diameter) into the proximal site of the distal fragment (**Figure 15.13**)
- Direct the K-wire distally towards the tips of the toes (or laterally). Shift the position of the drill from the proximal to the distal end of the toe. After displacement and rotation of the metatarsal head, the K-wire is oriented towards the medullary canal of the proximal fragment by means of a grooved probe. It is important to follow the longitudinal direction without dorsal or plantar deviation in order to maintain the new alignment (**Figure 15.14**)
- Remove the medial border of the proximal fragment with a Luer rongeur

Closure

- Wash the site abundantly to remove any bone debris

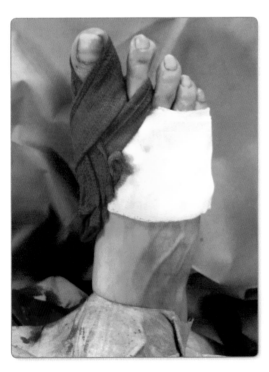

Figure 15.11 Imbricated gauzes to maintain the corrected axis (minimally invasive technique).

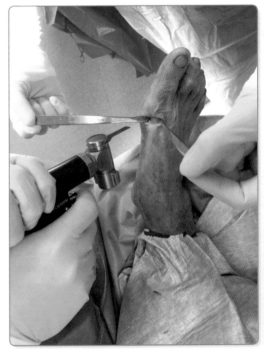

Figure 15.12 Bone exposure for the subcapital osteotomy.

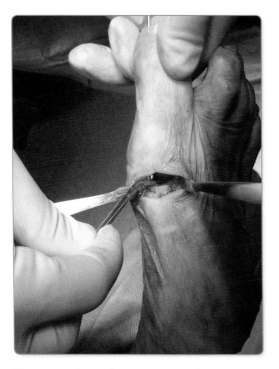

Figure 15.13 The Kirschner-wire is inserted using a guide.

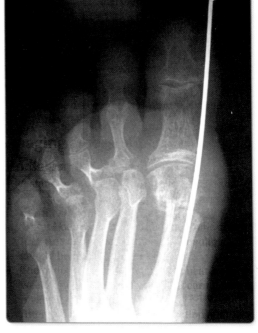

Figure 15.14 Radiographic image: the Kirschner-wire positioned and a new mechanical axis obtained.

- Suture the subcutaneous incision
- Soft tissue infiltration with ropivacaine around the osteotomy sites is advisable
- The foot is enclosed in multiple layers of sterile gauzes, protecting the protruding end of the K-wire
- A final elastic bandage is applied

Postoperative management

- After definitive radiographs the patient can be discharged either the same day or the day following surgery
- For 5 weeks after surgery, patients undergoing minimally invasive as well as an open procedure need to ambulate using a postoperative shoe (talus or Barouk shoe)
- Bleeding usually stops within 24 hours after surgery. The dressing of the surgical wound is changed on a weekly basis, using the same

procedure described above, both for the MIS and the Bosch/SERI surgical procedures. In case of the MIS technique, the gauze will be dry the 2nd week after surgery
- At 2 weeks following the MIS, a silicone spacer is applied between the first and the second toes for about 40 days
- At 6 weeks after surgery:
  - A plain radiograph is performed both for the MIS and Bosch/SERI techniques
  - The K-wire applied during the Bosch/SERI surgery is removed
  - The special postoperative shoe is abandoned and a shoe with a firm sole and soft upper is allowed
- Further radiologic evaluation is performed 3 months postoperatively (**Figure 15.15**)
- Two months after surgery, the clinician may recommend functional rehabilitation as well as passive and active mobilization in case of stiffness of the first MTP joint

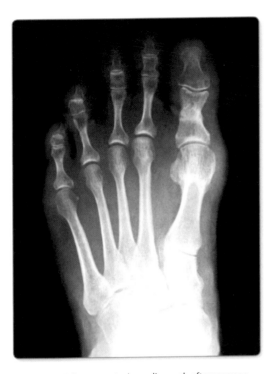

Figure 15.15 Anteroposterior radiograph after surgery.

Outpatient follow-up

- Bleeding: it can bleed inside the dressing after this surgery. You do not need to replace it
- Infection: this is the biggest complication in this surgery. We administer antibiotics perioperatively
- Delayed or nonunion: when the bone does not grow across the osteotomy
- Stiffness: the big toe is always stiff because of scar tissue
- Continuing symptoms: 80% of patients are satisfied, but some have pain due to scarring, and/or delayed union

Further reading

Bosch P, Wanke S, Legenstein R. Hallux valgus correction by the method of Bosch: a new technique with a seven-to-ten-year follow up. Foot Ankle Clin 2005; 5:485–498.

De Prado M. Complicaciones de la cirugia percutanea en el Hallux valgus. XII reunion anual de la SO.MA.C.OT. Madrid: 24-25 Mayo, 2001.

Giannini s, Ceccarelli F, Bevoni R, et al. Hallux valgus surgery: the minimally invasive bunion correction. Tech Foot Ankle Surg 2003; 2:11–20.

Sanna P, Ruiu GA. Percutaneous distal osteotomy of the first metatarsal (PDO) for the surgical treatment of Hallux valgus. Chir Organi Mov 2005; 90:365–369.

Surgical treatment for osteochondrosis of the second metatarsal head (Freiberg or Köhler II disease)

Indications

- The etiology of osteochondrosis is still unknown. The disorder arises in the period of maximum growth, occurring at skeletal sites where there is a nucleus of cancellous bone surrounded by cartilage
- Pathologically, it is characterized by the presence of aseptic necrosis, and radiographs show sequential stages of fragmentation and reconstruction of the bone nucleus (**Figure 16.1**)
- The final outcome may be a full recovery or alternatively an epiphyseal, metaphyseal, or apophyseal deformity according to the site of the lesion
- Freiberg's disease is the only osteochondrosis that occurs with greater frequency in the female sex, with a ratio of 5:1
- All the metatarsal heads may be affected, but the second and third metatarsal heads are more frequently involved

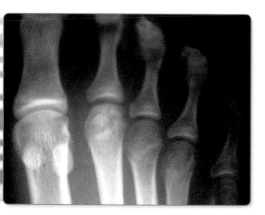

Figure 16.1 Radiograph showing fragmentation and reconstruction of the bone nucleus.

- Initial treatment involves no weight bearing on the affected area for 3–4 weeks. This is generally sufficient to achieve healing. However, in more advanced stages, when the articular surface is already partially compromised, surgical therapy may be required
- Surgery has been described involving a dorsiflexion osteotomy of the metatarsal head, described by Gauthier. In the more advanced stages an osteotomy alone may be insufficient, thus making arthroplasty with a periosteal strip an alternative treatment option

Preoperative assessment

Clinical assessment

- In the acute phase patients predominantly present with continuous pain in the affected metatarsal head
- On examination, the affected metatarsophalangeal joint has a restricted range of motion
- In adults particularly, pain may not present until late in the disease process or may be due to the presence of metatarsalgia

Imaging assessment

- Radiographs initially show flattening and fragmentation of the involved metatarsal head, which are characteristic
- Later in the disease process, the head and metaphyseal part of the affected metatarsal appear progressively deformed and enlarged (**Figure 16.2**)
- Typically, there is central flattening of the head with peripheral hyperostosis. Sometimes loose necrotic fragments may be evident

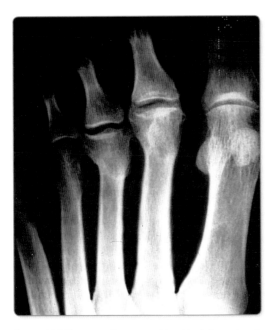

Figure 16.2 The second metatarsal head is deformed and enlarged.

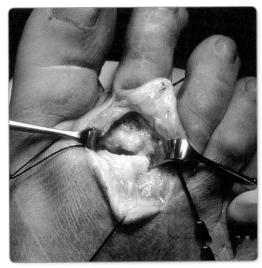

Figure 16.3 Reduction of joint space in addition to degeneration at the base of the proximal phalanx.

- In later stages of the disease, there is a reduction of the joint space and resulting structural and joint degeneration, also at the base of the phalanx (**Figure 16.3**)

Timing for surgery

- Surgery is predominantly reserved for cases in the advanced stages of the disease as in the early stages a period of nonweight bearing may be all that is required for resolution of the symptoms
- As the disease progresses but the joint surface is still partially preserved, removal of the loose fragments, synovectomy, and osteotomy as described by Gautier are indicated
- In the final stages of the disease, where there is marked articular destruction, surgical treatment in the form of the plastic flap of periosteum (as described below) may be required

Surgical preparation

Surgical equipment

For this procedure, the following instruments are required:

- Scalpel blades
- Scissors
- Klemmer forceps
- Motorized blades
- Sharp osteotomes
- Motorized rotary cutter (burr)
- Retractors and levers
- Kit for pull-out

Equipment positioning

- All instruments required for surgery are placed on a small sterile tray in front of the foot to be operated on

Patient positioning

- The patient is placed in the supine position
- The surgical field is prepared above the knee

Further preparation

- A tourniquet is applied above the knee for no more than 2 hours

Surgical technique

Exposure

- Metatarsophalangeal joint preparation:
  - A longitudinal S-shaped incision is carried out over the metatarsophalangeal joint (**Figure 16.4**)

- Once the joint capsule is exposed, a wide exposure is then carried out, with a subsequent capsulotomy, removing any loose articular bodies (**Figure 16.5**)
- The metatarsal head is now exposed and is prepared using a small ronguer or cutter (**Figure 16.6**)
- The hyperostosis is removed, along with the cartilage surface, followed by spherical remodeling (**Figure 16.7**)
- With hyperflexion of the toe, the base of the proximal phalanx is exposed; this is also prepared by removing any residual cartilage
- Graft harvesting:
  - A pretibial incision of about 10 cm in length is made below the anterior tibial tuberosity (**Figure 16.8**)

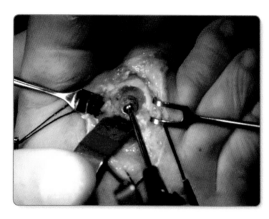

Figure 16.6 Preparation of the metatarsal head.

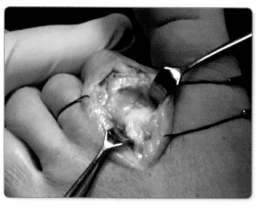

Figure 16.4 Surgical approach to the metatarsophalangeal joint with a longitudinal S-shaped incision.

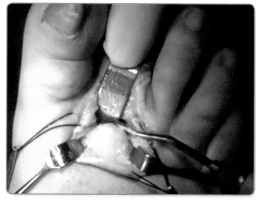

Figure 16.7 Spherical remodeling of the metatarsal head.

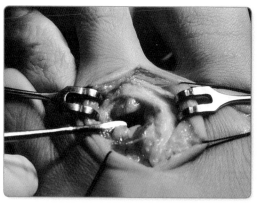

Figure 16.5 Removing any loose articular bodies.

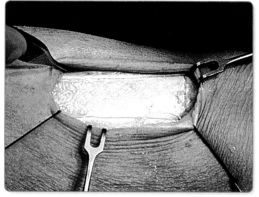

Figure 16.8 Pretibial incision for removing a periostal strip.

- The periosteal plane is revealed and a strip of about 8 cm × 2 cm is removed, which is loaded onto threads of absorbable suture with ethilon at the four corners and centrally on opposite sides (**Figure 16.9**)
- Graft interposition:
  - Returning to the metatarsophalangeal joint, the central threads, loaded on a needle, are passed through the sides of the joint and anchored on the plantar side onto a 'pull-out', placing the strip between the two joint heads (**Figure 16.10**); the strip therefore covers the joint surfaces with its deep side, while its surface layer is counterposed to constitute the neoarticular surfaces

- The dorsal parts of the strip, distal and proximal, are repacked and anchored on dorsal structure like periostium in order to completely cover the two articular heads (**Figure 16.11**)

Possible perioperative complications

- This approach is relatively safe and free from damage to the neurovascular structures
- Iatrogenic lesions of the extensor tendons may occur, which are repairable
- In some cases the remodeling of the joint can cause further destruction of the metatarsal head

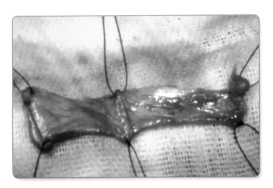

Figure 16.9 Loading the periostal strip at the four corners and centrally opposed sides.

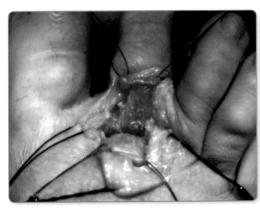

Figure 16.11 The dorsal parts of the strip, distal and proximal, are replaced and anchored in order to completely cover the two articular heads.

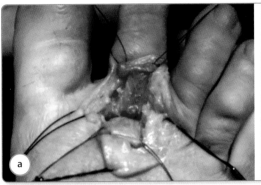

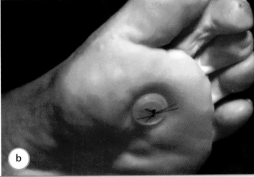

Figure 16.10 (a) Placing the strip betwin the two joint heads. (b) The plantar 'pull-out'.

Closure

- Suture for layers: adsorbable vicryl for subcutaneous layer and vicryl rapid for the skin
- Dressing with jelonet and imbricated
- Bandage

Postoperative management

- Nonweight bearing for 2 weeks: active and passive mobilization from the 10th day

- From 2 weeks, gradual weight bearing with postoperative shoes
- Removal of the pull-out after 6 weeks

Outpatient follow-up

- Weekly review for the first month until full weight bearing is resumed
- Regular analgesia for the first week
- Stitch removal at 2 weeks
- Monthly outpatient review until 1 year following the surgery

Further reading

Pisani G. Trattato di chirurgia del piede, 3rd edn. Torino: Edizioni Minerva Medica, 2004.

Parino E, Pisani PC, Milano L. Artroplastica per interposizione di periostio delle metatarso falangee esterne. Primi risultati a distanza. Chirurgia Del Piede 2002; 26:1–8.

Indications

- Achilles tendon disorders are divided into specific pathologies:
  - Paratenonitis
  - Tendinosis caused by partial ruptures
  - Paratenonitis and tendinosis, resulting from tendon overuse degeneration, partial tears or tendon calcifications
- Possible differential diagnoses of Achilles tendonitis/tendinosis are:
  - Partial rupture of the Achilles tendon
  - Retrocalcaneal bursitis
  - Insertional tendonitis
  - Subcutaneous Achilles tendon bursitis
  - Haglund's deformity
  - Calcaneal apophysitis
  - Calcaneal exostosis
- Achilles tendonitis can be divided into acute (symptoms duration less than 2 weeks), subacute (between 3 and 6 weeks), and chronic (more than 6 weeks) (El Hawary, 1997)
- Puddu published a detailed classification scheme of Achilles tendon disorders, on the basis of clinical and anatomic-pathologic findings (Puddu, 1976). The etiology may be also relevant when differentiating Achilles tendon pathologies. Many classification systems have been developed (van Dijk, 2011)
- Surgical treatment is recommended for patients who aim to resume physical activity who have been recalcitrant to nonoperative management

Contraindications

- Achilles tendon rupture
- Presence of tendon calcifications which may require excision of the calcified tissue and tendon repair

Preoperative assessment

Clinical assessment

Clinical presentation

- Some clinical aspects can vary according to the anatomic structures involved:
- When paratenonitis is present:
  - A crepitus may be heard as the tendon tries to glide within the inflamed paratenon, and pain arises during physical activity
  - The tendon is diffusely swollen
  - Usually, there is palpable tenderness on both sides of the tendon
  - Some nodules may possibly develop within the paratenon, leading subsequently to hypertrophy and connective tissue proliferation
- When tendinosis is present:
  - Symptoms arise gradually but are well localized within the middle third of the tendon
  - An inflammatory nodule may develop on the medial side of the tendon, the most hypovascular zone, which is also subject to the highest eccentric stresses
  - A localized medial thickening of the tendon is present
- If the degenerative process is extensive after repetitive partial ruptures, the tendon may appear elongated and its function decreased
- The Achilles tendon is exposed to high tensions and forces secondary to locomotion. An abnormal subtalar motion may overstress the tendon. During walking, jumping, and running activities both the gastrocnemius and the soleus muscles act as main plantar flexors via the Achilles tendon
- Achilles tendon injuries typically concern athletes, in particular runners

- In runners, the most common causes of Achilles tendon lesions are training mistakes, such as improper warm-ups, a sudden increase in workout intensity levels, excessive hill running, as well as changes in the contact with the ground surface (Schepsis et al, 2002)
- A cavus foot or a flat foot with hyperpronation may be a predisposing factor for Achilles tendon injuries

Physical examination

- Physical examination findings depend on the changes within the paratenon
- Insertional and noninsertional tendinopathy should be differentiated
- Lower extremity alignment should be observed in the standing position
- Both the ankle and the subtalar joint are assessed evaluating the range of motion. Plantarflexion and passive dorsiflexion are usually reduced
- The Thompson test is not diagnostic, unless a tendon rupture is present
- Peritendinous fibrous adhesions and thickening of the paratenon may be present, with the development of crepitus during fast up-and-down movements
- The clinician should palpate the tendon searching for nodules, fusiform swelling, and partial or complete defects

Imaging assessment

- Plain radiographs are rarely useful, due to the predominant presence of soft tissue injuries. However, they may help to evaluate the incidence of tendon ossification in cases of long-standing tendinosis
- Sonography is widely used. It is less expensive than MRI and allows a dynamic assessment. Focal hypoechoic intratendinous areas, localized tendon swelling, and thickening as well as discontinuity of tendon fibers are the main ultrasonographic findings. In chronic Achilles tendinopathy, peritendinous adhesions may be identified as a thickening of the hypoechoic paratenon with poorly defined borders (Reddy, 2009)
- However, it is an examiner-dependent technique and its reliability mainly depends on the experience of the operator
- MRI is outstanding in the preoperative assessment of Achilles tendon injuries. It is extremely sensitive to pathologic changes

within the tendon itself; (**Figure 17.1**) however, it may be less reliable in cases of thickening and fibrosis of the paratenon
- Achilles tendon tears usually occur 2–6 cm from its insertion. If they develop more proximally, then the musculotendinous junction together with the medial head of the gastrocnemius muscle are involved, as the presence of fluid on axial images shows. The edema within the muscle fibers may be diagnostic of a strain injury. The Achilles tendon fat pad presents thin septa and vessels (Del Buono, 2013)

Timing for surgery

- Surgery takes place after failure of conservative treatment
- The patient must have his maximal range of ankle movement

Surgical preparation

Special surgical considerations

- A thickened plantaris tendon located closely to the medial side of the Achilles tendon may

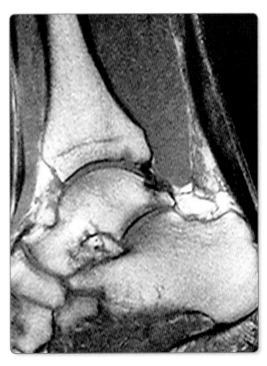

Figure 17.1 MRI showing thickening of the Achilles tendon.

occur in patients with chronic tendinosis. Since it may contribute to pain, surgical resection should be considered (Lui, 2013)
- Every surgical step must contribute to debulking the tendon and relieving adhesions
- The region 2–6 cm proximal to the Achilles insertion is prone to repetitive traumas in the so-called 'watershed region' (Kader, 2002)

Surgical equipment

Arthroscopic equipment (Figure 17.2)
- Arthroscope
- Light source and cables
- Camera system and monitor
- Arthroscopic probe (hook)
- Arthroscopic punches (basket forceps)
- Arthroscopic grasper
- Motorized ahaver
- Radio frequencies
- Arthroscopic burr

Equipment positioning
- The arthroscopic tower is positioned on the opposite side of the ankle, at the level of the patient's contralateral hip

Patient positioning
- The patient is placed in the prone position
- The contralateral leg is abducted, in order not to interfere with the operating field
- The feet are positioned just at the edge of the operating table, both to ensure a neutral position of the ankle and to allow a full range of motion during the surgical procedure
- The patient receives a single dose of intravenous antibiotics

- Anesthesia may be local, spinal, or general in specific cases according to the anesthesiologist's evaluation
- If local anesthetic is used, it is injected medially and laterally to the Achilles tendon (**Figure 17.3**)
- A tourniquet may be positioned on the ipsilateral thigh
- Inflate the tourniquet to 110 mmHg above the mean arterial pressure

Surgical technique

Achilles tendoscopy
- Posteromedial and posterolateral portals are made along the margins of the Achilles tendon, near its insertion on the calcaneus or at the musculo-tendinous junction (**Figure 17.4**)
- The subcutaneous space is inflated with 0.9% saline solution

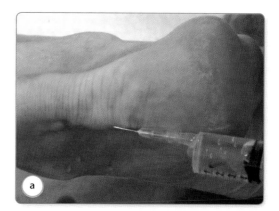

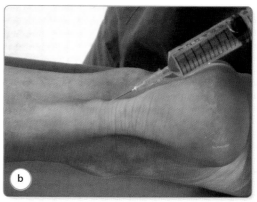

Figure 17.3 Local anesthesia: (a) medial and (b) lateral sides injected.

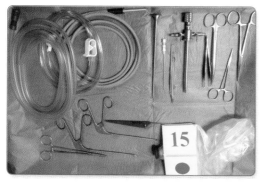

Figure 17.2 Complete arthroscopic set.

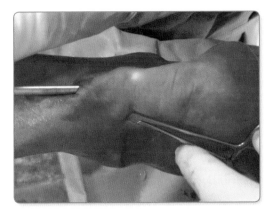

Figure 17.4 The operative portal is established under arthroscopic accessory view.

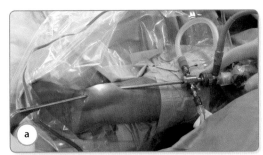

a

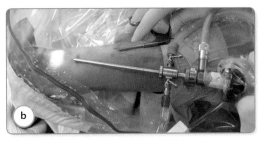

b

Figure 17.6 (a, b) Depending on the pathology, the operative portal may be selected where needed and moved distally (a) or proximally (b).

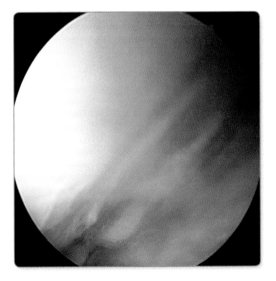

Figure 17.5 Endoscopic view of the Achilles paratenon.

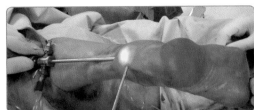

Figure 17.7 Paratenon dissection.

- The whole length of the tendon may be observed (**Figure 17.5**)
- Depending on the pathology, the operative portal is selected where needed (**Figure 17.6a** and **17.6b**)

Tissue dissection

- The cleavage plane between the tendon and the deep scar tissue is dissected using an arthroscopic shaver or a basket (**Figures 17.7–17.9**)
- The plantaris tendon is inspected and may be resected in order to avoid additional fibrosis

and restriction of the ankle range of motion (Lui, 2013)

- If necessary, longitudinal tenotomies may be performed along the longitudinal axis of the tendon, removing areas of tissue degeneration (Young et al, 2013)

Debridement

- Adhesions may be released with a shaver and freed from the surface of the Achilles tendon or dissected using a basket
- Debridement may be extended to the flexor hallucis longus to completely remove the deep scar tissue

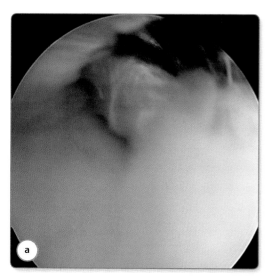

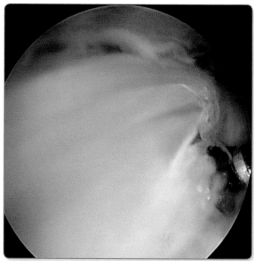

Figure 17.9 Achilles tendon free after tenolysis.

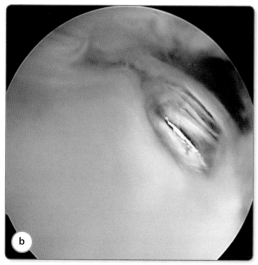

Figure 17.8 (a, b) Endoscopic view: the paratenon is dissected with a basket.

- If further release is necessary, the tenolysis can be extended to the dorsal side of the Achilles tendon

Possible perioperative complications

- Although arthroscopy is usually a safe surgical technique, it is important not to damage the neurovascular structures, particularly the sural nerve and the lateral calcaneal branch of the sural nerve (Morag, 2003)
- The tibialis posterior neurovascular bundle and the medial calcaneal branch of the tibial nerve lie relatively far from the surgical site

Closure

- Before the wound is closed, it is important to perform hyper-plantarflexion and dorsiflexion of the foot, in order to find any additional adhesions around the tendon
- Close the portal sites with 2-0 absorbable sutures
- Apply a compression dressing holding the foot in slight equinus

Postoperative management

Postoperative regimen

- 1 day postoperatively: Active and passive range of motion exercises may be started
- First 3 weeks postoperatively: Partial weight bearing is allowed; after this period full weight bearing is permitted
- Echographic evaluations may be used to stage the postoperative healing process (**Figure 17.10**)
- Once symptom-free, the patient can gradually resume their daily and sporting activities

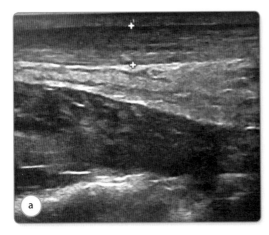 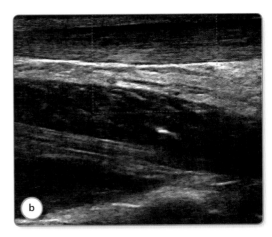

Figure 17.10 (a, b) Echographic evaluation 3 months after surgery. Picture (a) shows normal Achilles tendon along its whole path. (b) No vascular spots are present.

Early-phase postoperative complications

- The arthroscopic technique offers the advantage of low morbidity, good scar healing, and a very low grade of postoperative complications

Outpatient follow-up

- Patients are assessed at 6-monthly intervals for 1 year and discharged at that stage
- Further outpatient review is only required if symptoms return or a new trauma occurs

Further reading

Del Buono A, Chan O, Maffulli N. Achilles tendon: functional anatomy and novel emerging models of imaging classification. Int Orthop 2013; 37:715–21.

El Hawary R, Stanish WD, Curwin SL. Rehabilitation of tendon injuries in sport. Sports Med 1997; 24:347–358.

Kader D, Saxena A, Movin T, et al. Achilles tendinopathy: some aspects of basic science and clinical management. Br J Sports Med. 2002; 36:239–249.

Lui TH. Endoscopic Achilles tenolysis for management of heel cord pain after repair of acute rupture of Achilles tendon. J Foot Ankle Surg 2013; 52:125–127.

Schepsis AA, Jones H, Haas AL. Achilles tendon disorders in athletes. Am J Sports Med 2002; 30:287–305.

Morag G, Maman E, Arbel R. Endoscopic Treatment of Hindfoot Pathology. Arthroscopy 2003; 19:E13.

Puddu G, Ippolito E, Postacchini F. A classification of Achilles tendon disease. Am J Sports Med 1976; 4:145–50.

Reddy SS, Pedowitz DI, Parekh SG, et al. Surgical Treatment for Chronic Disease and Disorders of the Achilles Tendon. J Am Acad Orthop Surg 2009; 17:3–14.

van Dijk CN, van Sterkenburg MN, Wiegerinck JI, et al. Terminology for Achilles tendon related disorders. Knee Surg Sports Traumatol Arthrosc 2011; 19:835–841.

Young JS, Sayana MK, Testa V, et al. Percutaneous longitudinal tenotomies for chronic Achilles tendinopathy. In: Maffulli N, Easley M (eds), Minimally invasive surgery for Achilles tendon disorders in clinical practice. New York: Springer Science & Business Media, 2013:55–58.

18 Repair of Achilles tendon subcutaneous rupture with mini open technique

Indications

Achilles tendon repair using a mini open technique is indicated in:

- Active patients of any age with a subcutaneous acute rupture of the Achilles tendon

Contraindications

Achilles tendon repair using a mini open technique is contraindicated in:

- Chronic, retracted Achilles tendon ruptures (use an open technique)
- Nonactive patients over 65 years of age (use conservative treatment)
- Patients with lower limb vascular disease, diabetes, and skin ulcers as they are candidates for conservative treatment

Preoperative assessment

Clinical assessment

Patient history

- Patients present with sudden pain in the affected leg. They often believe that they have been kicked in the back of the leg
- Despite the typical presentation, it is common that a rupture is not diagnosed in the emergency room
- Physical examination may reveal a gap between the two stumps of the torn tendon
- The Thompson test ('calf squeeze test') is the diagnostic tool sufficient to make the diagnosis of tendon rupture: when squeezing the muscular part of the calf with the patient in the prone position, plantarflexion is absent when the tendon is ruptured
- Relevant lower limb vascular disease and skin ulcers should be considered in decision-making progress between conservative and surgical treatment

Imaging assessment

- Clinical examination is often sufficient to make the diagnosis of rupture of the Achilles tendon
- Ultrasonography or MRI can provide an additional contribution to the clinical diagnosis
- Not infrequently, the execution of ultrasonography and MRI examinations with doubtful answers can lead to an avoidable delay of surgical treatment

Ultrasonography

- If the tendon is torn, this may show an acoustic vacuum with thick, irregular edges
- The absence of a visible, clear interruption of tendon fibers can lead to misdiagnosis of a complete rupture

Magnetic resonance imaging (MRI)

- A complete rupture of the Achilles tendon is identified as a disruption of the signal within the tendon on T1-weighted images
- Increased signal intensity demonstrates edema and hemorrhage in T2-weighted images

Timing for surgery

- Surgery should take place if possible in the immediate period following the rupture
- Particular attention should be paid to patients with vascular disorders that could, especially in elderly patients, cause skin problems and blisters. In these cases it is always possible to consider nonoperative treatment with a dorsal splint

Surgical preparation

Surgical equipment

- Soft tissue surgical instrumentation and two Kirschner (K) wires that can be bent by the surgeon (**Figure 18.1**)

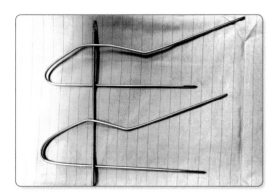

Figure 18.1 Two curved Kirschner (K)-wires are prepared, together with an isolated K-wire, to ensure subcutaneous passage of the suture in the Achilles tendon.

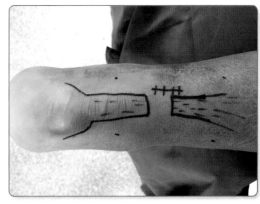

Figure 18.2 A longitudinal 2 cm paramedian incision is made a few millimeters proximal to the point of the rupture of the tendon.

- One slotted K-wire
- Absorbable 2.0 sutures
- Free needles

Equipment positioning

- Surgeon stands at the end of the operating table, with the assistant surgeon standing on the left and the scrub nurse on the right

Patient positioning

- A tourniquet is applied to the upper thigh with the patient in the supine position
- The patient is then placed prone with the ankle placed on a padded soft foot bar at the end of the operating table, in order to allow ankle plantar-and dorsi flexion
- Careful attention must be paid to the padding at the level of the iliac crests and chest

Surgical technique

- Inflate the tourniquet to 350 mmHg
- Exsanguinate the limb before making the first incision

Exposure

- A longitudinal paramedian incision 2 cm in length is made a few millimeters proximal to the palpable tendon gap (**Figure 18.2**)
- A longitudinal incision of the fascia and paratenon is performed, freeing the proximal (**Figure 18.3a**) and distal (**Figure 18.3b**) margins of the tendon stumps from skin adhesions

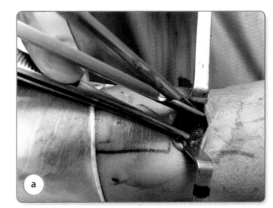

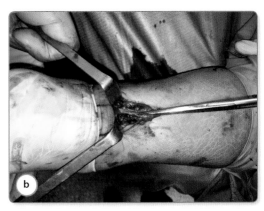

Figure 18.3 After the longitudinal incision of the skin and the paratenon has been made, it is necessary to free the proximal (a) and distal (b) margins of the tendon stumps from skin adhesions.

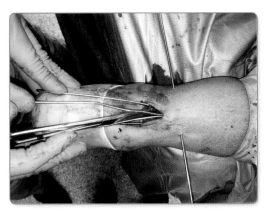

Figure 18.4 Two 2.0 mm curved Kirschner (K) wire suture guides are inserted medially and laterally to the proximal tendon stump. An isolated K-wire threaded with an absorbable 2.0 suture is then passed transversely through the skin, the intact tendon, and the apertures of the suture guides.

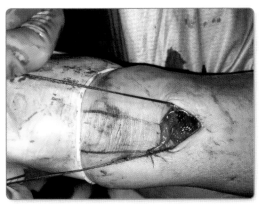

Figure 18.5 The Kirschner wires are retracted from the skin incision, recovering the wires introduced in to the proximal tendon stump.

Tendon repair

- The space between the subcutaneous tissue and the paratenon is demarcated using blunt dissection
- Two 2.0 mm curved K-wire suture guides are inserted medially and laterally to the proximal tendon stump. A long, straight needle or isolated K-wire threaded with an absorbable 2.0 suture is then passed transversely through the skin, the intact tendon, and the apertures of the suture guides (**Figure 18.4**)
- The K-wires are retracted from the skin incision, recovering the wires introduced in to the proximal tendon stump (**Figure 18.5**). The same surgical step is carried out for the distal tendon stump (**Figures 18.6–18.8**), facilitating the sliding of the tendon and accentuating the plantarflexion of the patient's foot
- Once both wires firmly anchor the proximal and distal stumps of the tendon and exit the skin incision (**Figure 18.9**), sutuing of the distal wires into the proximal tendon, and of the proximal wires into the distal tendon, is performed (**Figure 18.10**) with the same wires in order to reinforce the suture before the threads are knotted (**Figure 18.11**)

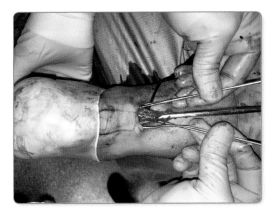

Figure 18.6 Kirschner wires are inserted medial and lateral to the distal stump of the Achilles tendon.

Possible perioperative complications

- The plantaris tendon is located close to the Achilles tendon in most cases
- Particular attention should be taken to nerve structures that can be entrapped during the suture passages, resulting in a postoperative skin dysesthesia or neuroma

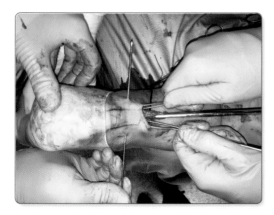

Figure 18.7 An isolated Kirschner wire is passed through the skin, the distal tendon, and the metallic suture guides.

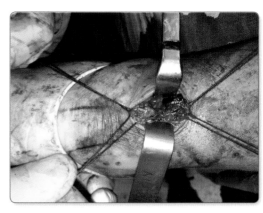

Figure 18.10 Suturing of the proximal wires to the distal tendon is performed in order to reinforce the tendon suture.

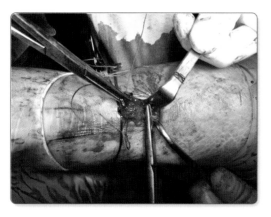

Figure 18.8 The distal suture is retracted, pulling the looped Kirschner wires through the surgical incision.

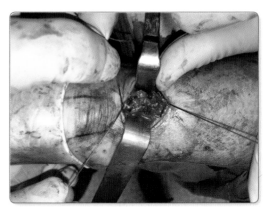

Figure 18.11 The wires emerging from the surgical incision are tied, with the ankle in slight plantarflexion, facilitating the final suture of the Achilles tendon.

- Skin adhesions can sometimes occur without real functional impairment but with esthetic concern, especially for women

Closure

- The paratenon should be sutured when possible with a 2.0 absorbable suture
- The subcutaneous layer is sutured with 2.0 absorbable sutures
- A continuous nylon or absorbable 2.0 skin suture is used for the skin (**Figure 18.12**)
- Standard analgesia is given
- A below-knee walker cast is applied at 15°, locked in plantar flexion
- The patient is nonweight bearing

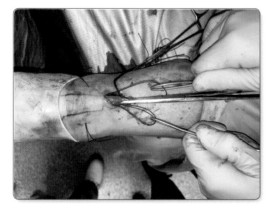

Figure 18.9 Suturing of the distal wires to the proximal stump is performed.

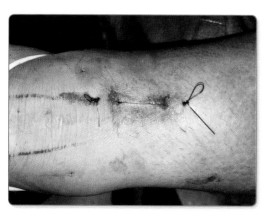

Figure 18.12 The skin layer is closed with an uninterrupted nylon 2.0 suture.

- 2 weeks postoperatively: stitches removed
- Hydrotherapy permitted as soon as the skin suture has healed
- 3 weeks postoperatively: gradual weight bearing allowed with crutches
- 5–6 weeks postoperatively: walker brace removed
- Graduated elastic stockings are applied after removal of the brace
- Exercises to recover musculo strength and elasticity of the musculo-tendinous unit
- Running allowed after 3 months and a full return to sport after 4–6 months

Postoperative management

- Day one: skin medication
- 1 week postoperatively: analgesia and a 0° locked walker brace

Further reading

De Carli A, Lanzetti RM, Ciompi A, et al. Can platelet-rich plasma have a role in Achilles tendon surgical repair? Knee Surg Sports Traumatol Arthrosc 2015 Mar 22: 1–7 [Epub ahead of print].

De Carli A, Vadalà A, Ciardini R, Iorio R, Ferretti A. Spontaneous Achilles tendon ruptures treated with a mini-open technique: clinical and functional evaluation. J Sports Med Phys Fitness 2009; 49:292–296.

Vadalà A, De Carli A, Vulpiani MC, et al. Clinical, functional and radiological results of Achilles tenorraphy surgically treated with mini-open technique. J Sports Med Phys Fitness 2012; 52:616–621.

Indications

- Calcific insertional Achilles tendonitis is an overuse syndrome resulting in enthesiopathy of the Achilles tendon
- Microtears within the tendon occur secondary to repetitive mechanical stress from overuse
- This causes collagen degeneration, fibrosis, and finally calcific metaplasia
- Predisposing conditions include Haglund's deformity and retrocalcaneal bursitis
- These conditions may exacerbate the condition by causing mechanical bony impingement and chemical irritation, respectively

Conservative management

- Initial management consists of a combination of the following:
  - Rest
  - Ice
  - Nonsteroidal anti-inflammatory medication
  - Activity and footwear modifications including pressure relief inserts
  - Physiotherapy and stretching exercises
  - Night splints
  - Ultrasound therapy
- If these measures fail, local injections can be given into the retrocalcaneal space. However, the concomitant use of local anesthetics and corticosteroids may further weaken the substance of the Achilles tendon and increase the risk of rupture
- While 90% of patients may respond temporarily to conservative treatment, many people have recurrent and persistent symptoms
- Failure of conservative measures is identified in the presence of ongoing pain and disability after appropriate conservative treatment in active patients
- Relative contraindications to surgical management are vascular or skin disorders affecting the lower limbs or patients who are very elderly or inactive

Preoperative assessment

Clinical assessment

Patient history

- Pain is localized to the posterior aspect of the calcaneus
- Pain is exacerbated when wearing rigid shoes, during the propulsive phase of the gait cycle, on ascending and descending stairs, and while running or participating in other sporting activities
- Patients may complain of weakness of the calf muscle. Initially the pain is intermittent but in severe cases it may be constant

Basic signs

- There may be a focal swelling around the posterior aspect of the calcaneus at the site of the Achilles tendon insertion
- An osseous bump may be located on direct palpation
- Pain may be reproduced on palpation, stretching the Achilles tendon, and loading with single or repeated heel rise exercises
- A swelling due to bursitis may be palpable anterior to the Achilles tendon

Physical examination

- A thorough assessment of the foot and ankle should include an examination of hindfoot alignment
- Attention should be paid to any calcaneovarus or valgus deformities
- The range of movement of the ankle and subtalar joints should be assessed, along with muscular power and a general examination of the foot and ankle

Imaging assessment

Radiographs

- The most useful plain radiographs should include the following views:

- Lateral weight-bearing images of the foot and ankle
- Saltzman view: anteroposterior weight-bearing radiograph of the ankle
- Axial view of the calcaneus
- Positive findings in calcific tendonitis include calcification at the Achilles tendon insertion visible on the lateral and axial views, and an abnormal prominence of the superoposterior aspect of the posterior tuberosity of the calcaneus
- On the Saltzman view attention should be paid to detecting any alteration of hindfoot alignment

Magnetic resonance imaging (MRI)

- MRI can assess the soft tissues in detail and give an overview of the condition of the Achilles tendon and the extension of the calcification; it can also confirm the presence of any associated bursitis
- On reviewing an MRI a bony spur is often evident at the posterior aspect of the calcaneus, corresponding to the Achilles tendon insertion
- Commonly, minor calcifications are located near the main ossification. Bursitis is generally present anterior to the Achilles tendon insertion
- There may be an area of bone bruising affecting the posterior tuberosity
- All these conditions are evident in the fat suppression series
- Another associated condition is an anomalous prominence of the superoposterior aspect of the calcaneus
- This may contribute to the impingement of the anterior part of the Achilles tendon

Timing for surgery

- Surgery should be carried out after a period of rehabilitation and muscular reinforcement
- Acute inflammation such as acute bursitis should be managed and resolved prior to surgery

Surgical preparation

Surgical equipment

- Standard surgical equipment for foot surgery including osteotomes, bone nibblers, and a power saw

Equipment positioning

- The surgeon should position themselves at the foot of the operating table with the assistant surgeon and the scrub nurse at either side of the operating table

Patient positioning

- The patient should undergo a spinal anesthetic or a peripheral nerve or ankle block, which can provide pain relief during and after surgery
- A high thigh tourniquet should be applied and the patient positioned prone with soft padding applied to prevent possible pressure sores (**Figure 19.1**)
- The operating table should be tilted into a slight anti-Trendelenburg position
- A cylindrical soft support is placed under the ankles to allow complete passive flexion and extension of the foot
- One dose of antibiotic prophylaxis should be administered prior to exsanguination of the limb and then inflation of the tourniquet to 300 mmHg

Surgical technique

- A 6–7 cm incision is made along the midline of the posterior aspect of the heel, starting 4–5 cm proximal to the Achilles tendon insertion and extending distally to the beginning of the plantar skin of the heel (**Figure 19.2**)
- A corresponding incision is made into the subcutaneous tissues down to the tendon (**Figure 19.3**). Care should be taken to create

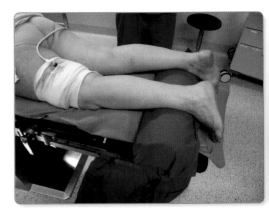

Figure 19.1 Patient positioning: prone position, tourniquet at the thigh, soft pad under the ankles.

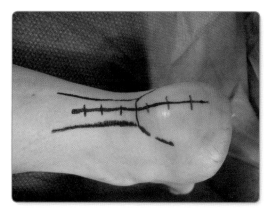

Figure 19.2 Skin incision along the midline of the Achilles tendon and the heel.

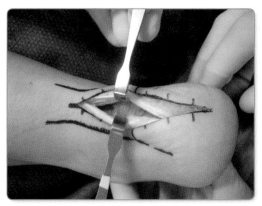

Figure 19.4 The paratenon and the Achilles tendon are divided longitudinally in the midline.

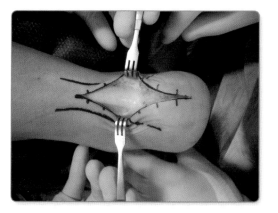

Figure 19.3 The skin and the subcutaneous tissues are retracted and the Achilles tendon is visualized.

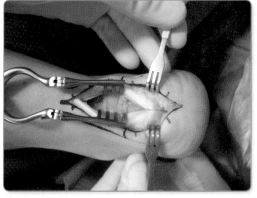

Figure 19.5 The two half tendons are separated and the postero-superior prominence of the calcaneum is visualized.

full-thickness skin flaps with diathermy to coagulate any small-vessel bleeding

- The paratenon and the Achilles tendon are incised longitudinally in the midline down to the bony insertion (**Figure 19.4**). The divided tendon is then spread laterally and medially using a self-retainer (**Figure 19.5**). The condition of the tendons is investigated in order to detect areas of degeneration
- The incision is extended distally along the same line on the posterior aspect of the calcaneus. At this point is easy to visualize the calcification of the insertion of the Achilles tendon
- The fibers of the tendon are carefully detached from the calcification and from the medial and

lateral aspects of the calcaneal tuberosity. At the distal part of the incision the periostium is detached from the calcaneus. At this stage the calcification is well isolated and visible (**Figure 19.6**). In general, approximately 50–70% of the Achilles tendon insertion is estimated to have been released during the debridement

- Within the split tendon the retrocalcanel bursa is isolated and excised. Usually, the bursa covers the posterior superior angle of the calcaneus and shows degenerative inflammatory and/or reactive fibrotic changes (**Figure 19.7**)
- After excision of the bursa the enlarged posterior superior border of the os calcis will come into view. Usually, the posterior aspect,

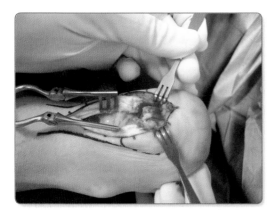

Figure 19.6 The insertions of the Achilles tendon are detached from the calcaneum.

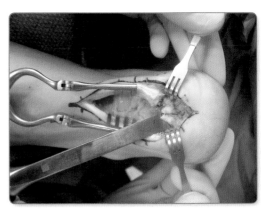

Figure 19.8 Resection of the insertional calcification.

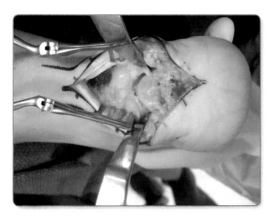

Figure 19.7 The insertional calcification is isolated.

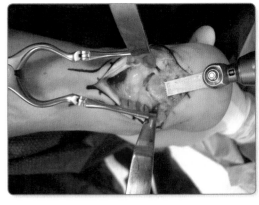

Figure 19.9 Resection of the postero-superior prominence of the calcaneum.

which corresponds to the retrocalcaneal bursa, is smooth while the superior border is prominent and irregular

- The insertional calcification is resected using an osteotome or an oscillating saw, and then any bony irregularity must be smoothed with bone nibblers (**Figure 19.8**)
- The prominent posterior superior aspect of the os calcis is also resected using an osteotome or oscillating saw. The resection is made from posterior to anterior starting from the tendon's insertion. The medial and lateral edges are also smoothed. For succesful results any Haglund's deformity must be adequately debrided and all sharp corners blunted. This will remove the mechanical impingement of the tendon that

results in degeneration. After the resection a thin film of bone wax is applied to the bony surface to avoid bleeding (**Figure 19.9**)

- The retrocalcaneal space is carefully irrigated and suctioned to remove any loose bony debris (**Figure 19.10**)
- At the end radiographs taken with an image intensifier or a mini C-arm are recommended. This is to check that the resection is adequate and to avoid leaving behind any bony prominences or small calcifications
- To reattach the tendon a 3.5 mm bony anchor with two sutures is placed in the calcaneus at the site of the resected calcification (**Figure 19.11**). The anchor should be directed either horizontally or slightly from plantar to dorsal

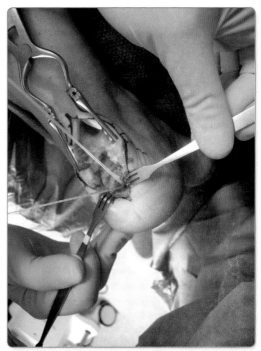

Figure 19.12 Checking the position of the sutures.

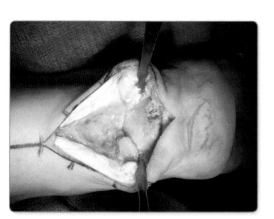

Figure 19.10 Posterior aspect of the heel after resections.

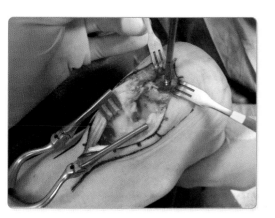

Figure 19.11 Positioning of a 3.5 mm bony anchor with two sutures.

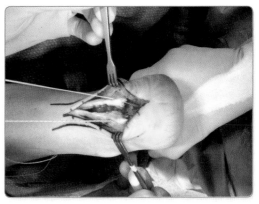

Figure 19.13 Two pairs of sutures are passed into each half tendon.

(**Figure 19.12**); the divided tendon is repaired with a single suture (**Figure 19.13**) and the suture is tied in a knot (**Figure 19.14**)
- The divided tendon is repaired with an absorbable 2.0 suture and the peritendon is repaired with an absorbable 3.0 suture (**Figure 19.15**)

- The foot is plantarflexed and dorsiflexed to check the stability of attachment of the Achilles tendon and to verify any last areas of impingement
- The tourniquet is than deflated and further hemostasis is performed if necessary
- Subcutaneous tissues are closed with 3.0 absorbable suture; the skin is closed in standard fashion

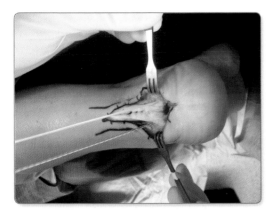

Figure 19.14 Final phase of the tendon reinsertion.

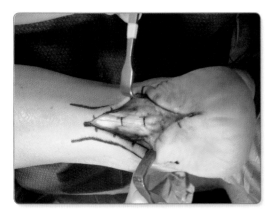

Figure 19.15 The Achilles tendon after the suture.

- A local anesthetic such as 0.25% Marcaine, without epinephrine (bupivacaine) is injected around the wound
- It is not necessary to place any surgical drains
- Only a simple dressing is required
- No rigid immobiliztation is advised

Options for surgical approach

- Various options for the surgical approach to the Achilles insertion have been described; these include a medial J-shaped incision, a lateral incision, a transverse incision, and a combination of medial and lateral approaches
- Because it extends to the central area of the tendon, the posterior midline central tendon-splitting approach was described to improve access to the tendon

- Medial, lateral, or combined approaches can cause difficulty in accessing and adequately debriding the tendon insertion. This can mean the calcific and scarred portion of the tendon might not be accessible without significant disruption of the remaining normal fibers of the tendon along its medial and lateral margins
- The central incision directly approaches the site of pathology without further damage to the uninvolved medial and lateral edges of the Achilles tendon, allowing the surgeon to treat the three major pathologic factors associated with this condition:
  1. Fibrosis and calcifications of the Achilles tendon
  2. Haglund's deformity
  3. Inflammation of the retrocalcaneal bursa

Options for surgical procedures

- In the presence of large calcifications which widely involve the insertion of the Achilles tendon or large areas of degeneration, a complete detachment of the Achilles tendon, its reattachment with suture anchors, and a proximal V–Y lengthening should be considered
- In such cases a 2–3 cm length of tendon is resected and a complete debridement of ossification and resection of prominence of the calcaneus is performed
- Following the tendon resection the distal tendon is inserted into a bony groove and reattached using four suture anchors
- If necessary the incision can be extended proximally and a V–Y lengthening performed at the musculotendinous junction to reduce tension
- The Achilles tendon can be supplemented using a graft of flexor hallucis longus tendon if the tendon is of poor quality

Possible perioperative complications

- Excessive or inadequate resection of the prominent posterosuperior aspect of the os calcis can occur if the bone cuts are sited incorrectly
- There may be poor fixation of the Achilles tendon, which can be supplemented with an additional bony anchor

- Thankfully, neurovascular complications are very rare using the posterior central approach. The most common injury is to the sural nerve or its branches during lateral approaches

Closure

- Subcutaneous tissues are closed with 3.0 absorbable suture; the skin is closed in standard fashion

Postoperative management

Postoperative regimen

- Analgesia with nonsteroidal anti-inflammatory drugs should be administered
- Postoperative lateral and axial radiographic views of the calcaneus should be performed
- Patients should remain on thromboembolic prevention for 6 weeks
- Patients should commence immediate mobilization without limitation. Passive motion exercises and isometric contractions should be performed to restore dorsiflexion of the ankle
- The patient should remain nonweight bearing for 3 weeks, followed by partially weight bearing with crutches for the next 3 weeks. Normal walking with full weight bearing can be resumed after a total of 6 weeks
- Swimming and cycling are encouraged after 3 weeks but other sporting activities are generally resumed 12 weeks after surgery

Early postoperative complications

- Swelling: this may be prevented with adequate elevation of the lower limb in the immediate postoperative period

- Wound dehiscence and/or tendon degeneration: the central approach decreases vascular compromise of the skin and of the Achilles tendon. The blood supply to the Achilles tendon is through its paratenon. Dissection medially or laterally, as performed with medial or lateral incisions, may impair blood flow to the tendon and lead to poor healing
- Pain at the site of the tendon insertion: it is very important to completely resect the insertional calcifications and to smooth carefully the edges of the resected area of the calcaneus. Using a medial or lateral approach may limit exposure and contribute to inadequate debridement
- Stiffness in flexion and/or extension: to prevent this complication early mobilization and rehabilitation are recommended
- Triceps surae weakness
- Risk of rupture or avulsion of the Achilles tendon (5%): the midline approach allows the surgeon to easily identify how much tendon has been debrided and to assess the stability of the Achilles tendon insertion
- Up to 50% of the tendon can be debrided safely. However, a failure to identify excessive debridement of the tendon will compromise the insertion site and may predispose it to rupture
- Usually, a fixation of the tendon with one anchor provides sufficient stability and allows immediate mobilization. If there has been excessive debridement of the insertion site the use of two anchors is recommended

Further reading

Kang S, Thordarson DB, Charlton TP. Insertional Achilles tendinitis and Haglund's deformity. Foot Ankle Int 2012; 33:487–491.

Kearney R, Costa ML. Insertional achilles tendinopathy management: a systematic review. Foot Ankle Int 2010; 31:689–694

Nunley JA, Ruskin G, Horst F. Long-term clinical outcomes following the central incision technique for insertional Achilles tendinopathy. Foot Ankle Int 2011; 32:850–855.

Roche AJ, Calder JD. Achilles tendinopathy: A review of the current concepts of treatment. Bone Joint J 2013; 95-B:1299–1307.

Treatment for chronic midportion Achilles tendinopathy: the soleus transfer technique

Indications

- Chronic midportion Achilles tendinopathy is an overuse pathology that typically occurs in middle-aged athletes (de Jonge et al, 2011), but can affect younger athletes too
- The main pathological feature is a fusiforme thickening of the midportion of the Achilles tendon. This thickening is caused by an internal area of ischemic degeneration
- The most common etiology is a failed healing response with haphazard proliferation of tenocytes, disruption of collagen fibers, and subsequent increase of the noncollagenous matrix, i.e. proteoglycans
- The thickening increases over time and the anatomic-pathologic symptoms worsen
- Physical activity triggers pain, which in turn makes such activity less feasible. Patients affected by advanced forms of the pathology experience pain when simply walking
- Physiotherapy should aim towards tendon reconstruction, but the persistence of symptoms and anatomo-pathology after six months of therapy, establishes the tendinopathy as chronic and conservative treatment will cease to be effective. At this point, surgery is necessary
- The affected portion is between 2 and 7 cm from the calcaneal insertion of the Achilles tendon
- There is usually an absence of any inflammatory response
- The rationale of soleus transfer is that it restores blood supply to an area of ischemic degeneration and thus facilitates tissue healing and regeneration. This surgical technique is indicated by Benazzo et al (2014) in the following situations:

  - Athletes of all ages
  - Patients with chronic midportion Achilles tendinopathy that is resistant to conservative treatments
  - Patients with symptoms after more than 4 months of conservative treatment
  - Patients complaining of pain during sport activities or during lengthy walks
  - Patients with pathologic findings on MRI

Preoperative assessment

Clinical assessment

Patient history

- Patients report pain at the beginning of, and after, sport activity
- Pain intensity is variable but is always localized at the midportion of the Achilles tendon
- Patients often experience pain during their first steps in the morning

Physical examination

- Examination reveals fusiform, hard thickening of the midportion tendon
- Palpation of this area reveals a localized nodule, which moves with the tendon during ankle movements, and is severely painful
- Chronic inflammation can afflict the peritenon, which in turn can thicken and thus increase pain

Imaging assessment

Ultrasonography

- Ultrasound detects increases in the diameter of the Achilles tendon midportion
- Sonography reveals focal alteration in tendon echotexture. It can also reveal peritenon thickening

- Doppler ultrasound typically fails to identify hypervascularization in the degenerative zone

Magnetic resonance imaging (MRI)

- Sagittal and coronal sections detect fusiform thickening of the midportion of the Achilles tendon, while the transverse sections reveal an increase in tendon diameter and a central mucoid degenerative area that is surrounded by approximately normal tissue
- The zone of ischemic degeneration is hyperintense on T1 and T2 MRI-weighted images. This is pathognomonic of tendinopathy
- In addition MRI is useful to assess the distance of the soleus myotendinous junction from the pathologic area of the tendon. This measurement allows an estimation of whether it is possible to implement this technique

Timing for surgery

- Recourse to surgery should only be taken after a minimum of 4 months physical therapy particularly focusing on eccentric strengthening, and produces no clinical improvement
- Patients should be advised in advance that they will undergo medium-to-long term postoperative therapy before they can return to sport, and that their daily life in the immediate postoperative phase will be subject to limitations

Surgical preparation

Surgical equipment

- Absorbable sutures are required to fix the soleus and repair the tendon incision

Equipment positioning

- The surgeon and assistant face one another across the foot of the table with the scrub nurse at the foot of the table

Patient positioning

- The patient should undergo a spinal anesthetic or a peripheral nerve or ankle block which can offer pain relief during and after surgery
- A high thigh tourniquet should be applied and the patient positioned prone with soft padding applied to prevent pressure sores

- The patient's feet should overhang the end of the operating table, with their ankles on top of a sandbag

Surgical technique

Exposure

- The initial step is to exsanguinate the limb and inflate the tourniquet to 320 mmHg, preferably with the patient in a supine position. The patient should then assume the prone position, prior to sterile field set up
- Following this, a longitudinal skin incision should be made at the lateral border of the Achilles tendon
- The incision should be long enough to permit good exposure of the distal fibers of the soleus
- Incise the peritenon and detach it from the tendon; the former is typically thicker than normal and adherent to the tendon
- From a frontal position, identify the distal portion of the soleus and, on the basis of naked eye evidence, assess whether it is possible to effect a transfer to the degenerative zone
- Care should be taken to identify and protect the sural nerve, which is then laterally divaricated

Soleus transfer preparation

- Blunt dissection should be used to identify a cylindrical bundle of the inferolateral portion of the soleus muscle
- The bundle is left attached distally (**Figure 20.1**). Later the proximal edge of the bundle will be incised, leaving the bundle long enough to rotate and cover the degenerated area of the tendon (**Figure 20.2**)

Tendon debridement

- A single central full-thickness longitudinal incision of the tendon is made where it crosses the degenerated midportion (**Figure 20.3**)
- Remove any internal degenerated tissue, the opacity of which will contrast the lustre of healthy tendon tissue. The consistency of degenerated tissue will also be malacic. Such tissue must be removed by scarification and/or longitudinal internal incisions on the tendon

Transfer positioning

- After measuring and proximally dividing the correct length of the soleus bundle, rotate the

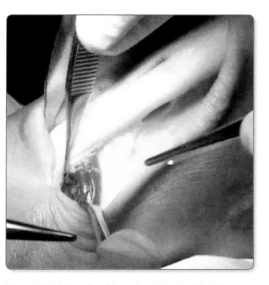

Figure 20.1 A bundle of the soleus is isolated by blunt dissection.

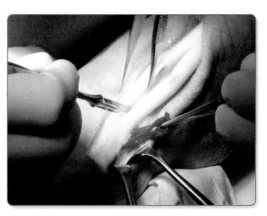

Figure 20.3 Full-thickness longitudinal incision of the tendon.

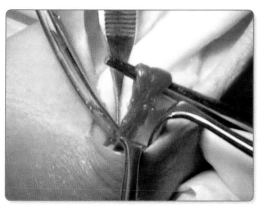

Figure 20.2 Detaching a bundle of correct length.

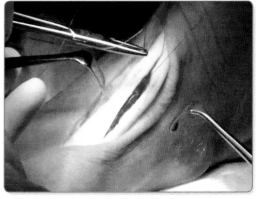

Figure 20.4 The transfer anchored distally with an absorbable suture.

bundle by 180° and place it inside the tenotomy
- Avoid twisting or excessive tension of the bundle, to prevent any interruption of the blood flow to the tendon
- Anchor the bundle's distal end and fix it to the internal portion of the tendon with thin reabsorbable suture (**Figure 20.4**)
- Care should be taken not to apply any traction to the soleus graft, to avoid ischemic damage of the muscle tissue
- Use only nonabsorbable sutures to reconnect the separated tendon; ensure you neither

constrain the muscular flap nor completely close the tendon
- Deflate the tourniquet and check the blood supply to the graft

Possible perioperative complications

- There may be an insufficient length of soleus muscle fibers to graft over the degenerated tendon area. This can occur if there is not a long enough muscle bundle (high soleus) or the bundle is divided to too short a length

- The salvage solution is to perform multiple tenotomies (Paavola et al, 2002)
- If the muscle bundle or its vascular supply is stripped, the salvage solution is multiple tenotomies

Closure

- No tendon or paratenon repair sutures are needed
- On the bases that bleeding is desirable, but hematoma is to be avoided, a small drain can be placed and left in situ for 24 hours
- The skin is closed with intradermal sutures and a simple dressing is applied
- Only a bandage should be applied; no immobilization is necessary

Postoperative management

- Patients are discharged on the first day after surgery, conditionally upon removal of the drain and ascertainment that bleeding and other complications are absent. Progressive passive mobilization of the ankle should be undertaken from the first postoperative day
- A light dressing should be applied for 2 weeks
- Weight bearing should be avoided for the first 3 weeks. Passive and active mobilization of

the ankle should be encouraged to prevent adhesions. Early isometric and isotonic exercises of the calf should be performed, and once the wound has healed hydrotherapy may be useful

- After 3 weeks, progressive weight bearing is allowed, to reach 100% in c. 15 days
- Further rehabilitation can commence 3 weeks postoperatively once the swelling has settled and a complete range of motion has returned
- The patient should then start to perform strengthening exercises first with open kinetic chain exercises, performed where the foot is free to move, and static proprioception training. This can be followed by close kinetic chain exercises, performed where the foot remains in constant contact with the ground or the base of a machine, aerobic training, progressive eccentric strengthening exercises, and dynamic proprioception activity
- Running may be allowed when the patient recovers a good strenghtening of the triceps surae at around 4 months. Initially, running should be on a flat surface

Outpatient follow-up

- Wound checks should be performed at 7 and 14 days
- Medications: NSAIDs; and thromboembolic prophylaxis should be given for 3 weeks
- There should be clinical and ultrasonography assessement at 2, 3, and 4 months postoperatively

Further reading

Benazzo F, Zanon G, Klersy C, Marullo M. Open surgical treatment for chronic midportion Achilles tendinopathy: faster recovery with the soleus fibres transfer technique. Knee Surg Sports Traumatol Arthrosc 2014 Sep 6 [epub ahead of print].

de Jonge S, van den Berg C, de Vos RJ, et al. Incidence of midportion Achilles tendinopathy in the general population, Br J Sports Med 2011; 45:1026–1028.

Paavola M, Kannus P, Orava S, et al. Surgical treatment for chronic Achilles tendinopathy: a prospective seven month follow up study. Br J Sports Med 2002; 36:178–182.

Retinaculum repair for recurrent peroneal tendon subluxation

Indications

- Surgery is indicated in the instance of ongoing pain and instability in active patients
- Instability may involve a sensation of the tendons 'popping' or 'jerking' over the lateral malleolus or the ankle giving way
- The injury is usually related to sporting activities such as skiing, soccer, rugby, basketball, tennis, and dancing

Contraindications to surgery

- Surgery may not be suitable for elderly and inactive patients or those with vascular or skin disorders affecting the lower limbs

Classification

The subluxation of peroneal tendons has been classified by Oden into four groups:

- *Group I*: avulsion of the superior retinaculum and of the periostium from the lateral aspect of the fibula. The peroneal tendons are subluxed anteriorly between the bone and the periosteum
- *Group II*: detachment of the superior retinaculum from the cartilaginous posterior edge of the fibula
- *Group III*: avulsion of the superior retinaculum from the fibula with an avulsion fracture of the posterior and/or lateral aspect. The peroneal tendons are often subluxed into the fracture
- *Group IV*: posterior rupture of the posterior retinaculum

Group I type lesions occur most commonly. The surgical technique that will be described is mainly applied to the treatment of group I lesions.

Preoperative assessment

Clinical assessment

Patient history

- Often an ankle sprain with inadequate treatment is reported
- The patient may report a sensation of lateral instability of the ankle
- In many cases there is giving way of the ankle combined with a snapping sensation over the lateral ankle
- In several cases mild pain is reported around the lateral malleolus
- In some cases the patient is able to spontaneously manipulate and sublux the peroneal tendons anteriorly and to reduce them with or without pain

Physical examination

- There may be swelling around the lateral malleolus
- On foot dorsiflexion and eversion the peroneal tendons sublux anteriorly over the lateral malleolus (**Figure 21.1**)
- There may be snapping and crepitus during active movements of the ankle, paticularly pronation–supination

Further physical assessment

- Overall stability of the ankle should be assessed
- Varus–equinus and anterior drawer stress tests should be performed
- The alignment of the hindfoot, range of movement of the ankle and subtalar joint, and muscular strength should be assessed
- There should be a general examination of the foot and ankle

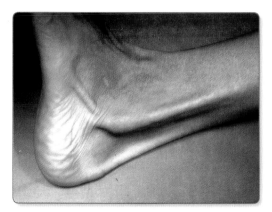

Figure 21.1 Dislocation of peroneal tendons during dorsiflexionand eversion movements.

Imaging assessment

Radiographs

- Lateral weight-bearing radiographs of the foot and ankle including Saltzman views should be taken. These images will evaluate the general morphology of the foot
- Anteroposterior and mortise views of the ankle may detect a possible avulsion fracture of the lateral aspect of the lateral malleolus

Magnetic resonance imaging (MRI)

The aim of MRI is to assess for the following problems:

- Avulsion of the retinaculum from the posterior edge of the fibula
- Possible direct visualization of the peroneal tendons in subluxation
- Degenerative conditions of the peroneal tendons such as longitudinal tears
- Any injury to the lateral ligaments of the ankle and the cartilage of the tibiotalar and talocalcaneal joints
- Abnormal morphology of the posterior fibular groove such as a flat or convex appearance
- Osseus lesions such as avulsion fractures (although for osseous problems CT is more sensitive than MRI)

Surgical preparation

Surgical equipment

- Standard surgical equipment for foot surgery including a power drill and saw

Patient positioning

- The patient should undergo a spinal anesthetic or a peripheral nerve or ankle block, which can offer pain relief during and after surgery
- A high thigh tourniquet should be applied and the patient positioned in the lateral decubitius position. The pelvis should be stabilized with a support on either side of it. The contralateral knee is flexed to 90°. Softs pads need to be applied to prevent possible pressure sores **(Figure 21.2)**
- One dose of antibiotic prophylaxis should be administered prior to inflation of the tourniquet to 300 mmHg

Surgical technique

- A 5 cm incision is made 15 mm posterior to the posterior edge of the lateral malleolus and curved anteriorly to the tip of the malleolus **(Figure 21.3)**
- Any traversing small vessels are coagulated
- The sural nerve is identified in the posterior and distal part of the incision and protected
- Next the peroneal sheath and the superior retinaculum are identified. Usually, the peroneal tendons can be subluxed anteriorly with gentle pressure or by holding the foot in dorsiflex and eversion
- The peroneal sheath and the superior retinaculum are incised longitudinally about 1 cm posterior to the edge of the lateral malleolus, distally to the tip of the fibula **(Figure 21.4)**

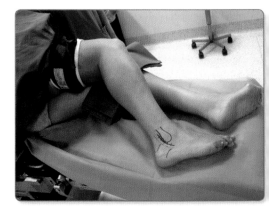

Figure 21.2 Patient positioning: lateral decubitus stabilized with lateral pad, tourniquet at the thigh.

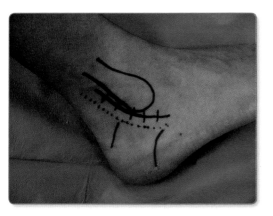

Figure 21.3 Skin incision.

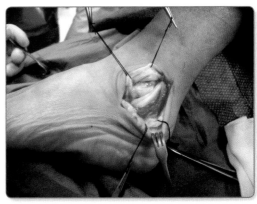

Figure 21.5 Avulsion of the superior retinaculum and of the periosteum from the lateral aspect of the fibula.

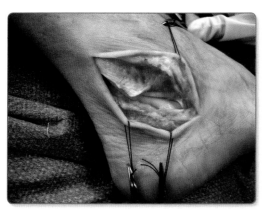

Figure 21.4 Incision of retinaculum.

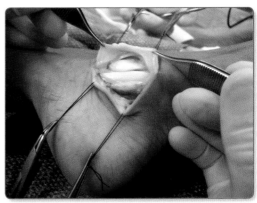

Figure 21.6 The detached superior reinaculum from the fibula.

- The peroneal tendons are examined in order to detect any longitudinal or partial tears
- If any tears are present they must be repaired using a strong absorbable suture
- The avulsion of the superior retinaculum and of the periosteum from the lateral aspect of the fibula is visualized (**Figure 21.5**)
- Usually, there is a large pocket with smooth surfaces into which the peroneal tendons can be subluxed (**Figure 21.6**)
- The ankle should be assessed for anterior subluxation of the peroneal tendons. The maneuver to assess for this is direct pressure on the tendons from posterior to anterior, or moving the foot into dorsiflexion and eversion
- The posterior fibular groove is examined. If the groove in congenitally shallow, flat, or

convex, techniques of deepening must be considered
- The two surfaces of the pocket of dislocation are debrided by excising any scarred or fibrous tissue. Particular attention should be paid to the area adjacent to the posterior edge of the fibula
- The most important step of the procedure is the fixation of the detached superior retinaculum and the periosteum to the posterior edge of the fibula (**Figure 21.7**)
- Three or four transverse parallel holes are drilled in the posterior edge of the fibula starting from the apex and running 3–4 cm proximally (**Figure 21.8**)
- A long-term absorbable 2.0 suture is passed from superficial to deep in the retinacular or

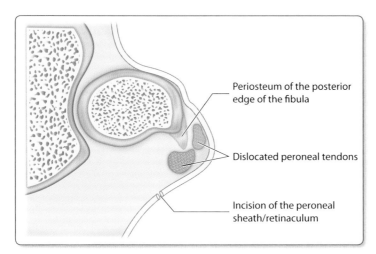

Figure 21.7 Cross section schema of the anatomy of the lesion.

Periosteum of the posterior edge of the fibula

Dislocated peroneal tendons

Incision of the peroneal sheath/retinaculum

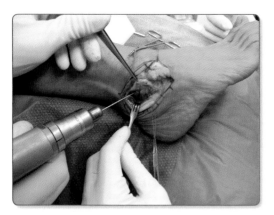

Figure 21.8 Bony tunnels are drilled in the posterior edge of the fibula.

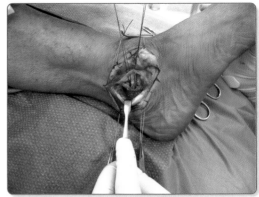

Figure 21.9 The detached flap of retinaculum is fixed to the fibula.

the periosteal flap. The suture is first passed through a drill hole, then passed in the opposite direction through an adjacent drill hole, and finally secured into the retinacular/periosteal flap (**Figure 21.9**)

- The suture should then be knotted tightly to push the flap against the bone and close the pocket into which the tendons have been subluxing. Three or four sutures are then passed using the same method to secure the detached retinaculum/periosteum (**Figure 21.10**)
- The sheath of peroneal tendon is closed with an absorbable 3.0 suture
- The foot is dorsiflexed and everted in order to check the stability of the tendons
- The tourniquet is deflated and any bleeding vessels are cauterized

Additional procedures

- Many techniques to deepen the posterior fibular groove have been described
- One of the most simple methods is to drill caudally from an entry point at the tip of the fibula
- The drill should be directed parallel and very close to the posterior cortex
- The drill hole is expanded with a 5 mm reamer and completed with a curette
- The posterior cortex is then gently struck with a smooth instrument to deepen the groove
- If a fracture of the posterior edge of the fibula occurs it must be fixed with mini-screw or absorbable pins
- An alternative technique is to use a rotary burr to deepen the grove in the posterior fibula

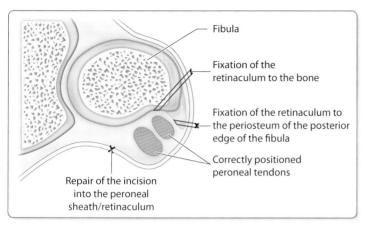

Figure 21.10 Cross section schema after the repair.

Labels on figure:
- Fibula
- Fixation of the retinaculum to the bone
- Fixation of the retinaculum to the periosteum of the posterior edge of the fibula
- Correctly positioned peroneal tendons
- Repair of the incision into the peroneal sheath/retinaculum

Possible perioperative complications

- If the fixation of the retinaculum/periosteal flap to the bone is inadequate, a bony anchor should be used to supplement the repair

Closure

- Subcutaneous tissues are closed with 3.0 absorbable suture
- The skin is closed in the standard fashion
- Local anesthetic such as 0.25% Marcaine without epinephrine (bupivacaine) is infiltrated around the wound
- No wound drains are required
- After application of a simple dressing the foot is placed in a below-knee cast or in a splint in a neutral position

Postoperative management

Postoperative regimen

- This should involve analgesia with nonsteroidal anti-inflammatory drugs

- Thromboembolic prevention should be given for 6 weeks. The belowknee cast or splint should be worn for 4 weeks
- The patient should be nonweight bearing for 4 weeks and then partially weight bearing with a bivalved orthosis for 2–3 weeks
- After removing the cast, mobilization and physiotherapy with passive and active movements, and isometric contractions should be commenced
- Normal walking with full weight bearing can be resumed after 6–7 weeks and sporting activities are generally resumed 12 weeks after operation

Early-phase postoperative complications

These can be summarized as follows:

- Swelling
- Recurrence of subluxation (5–10%)
- Wound dehiscence
- Pain along the peroneal tendons
- Stiffness in ankle flexion and/or extension
- Peroneal muscle weakness

Further reading

Cho J, Kim JY, Song DG, Lee WC. Comparison of Outcome After Retinaculum Repair With and Without Fibular Groove Deepening for Recurrent Dislocation of the Peroneal Tendons. Foot Ankle Int 2014; 35:683–689.

Ferran NA, Oliva F, Maffulli N. Recurrent subluxation of the peroneal tendons. Sports Med 2006; 36:839–846.

Raikin SM. Intrasheath subluxation of the peroneal tendons. Surgical technique. J Bone Joint Surg Am 2009; 91:146–155.

Saxena A, Ewen B. Peroneal subluxation: surgical results in 31 athletic patients. J Foot Ankle Surg 2010; 49:238–241.

Surgical treatment of peroneal tendon lesions

Indications

Surgical treatment of peroneal tendon lesions is indicated in the presence of the following:

- Resistant symptoms despite conservative management including anti-inflammatory medications, lateral heel wedge, bracing, and physiotherapy
- Severe posterolateral ankle pain
- Swelling along the peroneal tendon sheath
- Instability with associated reduced function
- A history of an ankle sprain that has never fully resolved

Preoperative assessment

Clinical assessment

- Basic signs of a peroneal tendon lesion include:
  - Swelling posterolaterally along the course of the tendons, and pain on palpation along the course of the tendons
  - Pain exacerbated by compression of the superior peroneal retinaculum as the patient actively everts the ankle (Sobel's sign)
  - There may be crepitus or popping of the tendons: Sobel et al described the peroneal compression test, which is used to assess for pain, crepitus, and 'popping' at the posterior edge of the distal fibula during forceful eversion and dorsiflexion of the ankle
  - Difficulty in maintaining stability on a single-stance heel rise, and retromalleolar pain on anterior drawer testing. There is also decreased peroneal muscle strength
- However, the peroneus tertius, extensor digitorum longus, and extensor hallucis longus provide some compensatory eversion function so absence of weakness on eversion does not rule out a peroneal tendon tear or rupture

- The signs and symptoms may be more severe in young or highly active patients, and some elderly patients may be completely asymptomatic

Physical examination

- Ankle and hindfoot malalignment is an important factor predisposing to peroneal lesions
- A cavovarus foot position may cause overloading of the peroneal tendons during activity, leading to tears
- In these cases, the peroneus longus tendon is most likely to be affected
- Peroneal tendon tears are frequently associated with other disorders, such as severe ankle sprains or chronic ankle instability
- Anatomic variations, including a shallow retromalleolar groove, a low-lying peroneus brevis muscle belly, a peroneus quartus muscle, and posterolateral fibular spurring, may predispose to a peroneal tendon lesion
- Longitudinal split tears of the peroneus brevis are usually found within the retromalleolar sulcus. Peroneus longus ruptures usually occur at the level of the cuboid, at the os peroneum, at the peroneal tubercle, or at the tip of the lateral malleolus

Imaging assessment

Radiographs

- Lateral weight-bearing radiographs of the foot and ankle including Saltzman views should be taken. Anteroposterior and mortise views of the ankle and dorsoplantar views of the foot are also required
- These radiographs are useful for evaluating acute osseous injuries, such as fractures of the calcaneus, lateral malleolus, or os peroneum. The os peroneum is normally located at the cuboid notch; fracture or migration of the os peroneum should alert the surgeon to the possibility of a peroneus longus tendon tear

- Chronic conditions can also be diagnosed, such as lateral ankle impingement, hypertrophy of the peroneal tubercle, spurring of the retromalleolar groove, and exostoses
- Alignment can be assessed on the lateral view of the foot using Meary's line and assessing the height of the fifth metatarsal relative to the first metatarsal

Magnetic resonance imaging (MRI)

- MRI is the standard method for evaluating tendon disorders due to its sensitivity in assessing soft tissues
- The axial views with the foot in slight plantarflexion are the most useful images for evaluating the peroneal tendons
- A peroneus brevis tear may appear as a C-shaped or bisected tendon or as an increased intratendinous T2-weighted signal
- A peroneus longus tear may demonstrate a linear or round area of increased signal within the tendon, marrow edema along the calcaneal wall, or a hypertrophic peroneal tubercle
- MRI is useful in excluding other differential diagnoses of chronic lateral ankle pain

Classification

- Transverse ruptures
  - Partial tears
  - Complete rupture
  - Peroneus brevis and peroneus longus or both
- Longitudinal ruptures
  - Grade I: an enlarged or flattened tendon without rupture
  - Grade II: partial ruptures
  - Grade III: complete longitudinal ruptures of less than 2 cm
  - Grade IV: complete longitudinal ruptures of more than 2 cm
  - Peroneus brevis and peroneus longus or both

Surgery

- Operative treatment of peroneal tendon lesions varies depending on the severity of the pathologic involvement
- Given that diagnosis of peroneal lesions is largely clinical, often the extent of the injury is not known before surgical exploration. The type of repair undertaken is therefore based on the surgical findings

Surgical preparation

Surgical equipment

- Normal surgical equipment for the foot including a power drill and saw

Equipment positioning

- The surgeon is positioned at the foot of the table behind the patient (i.e. on the affected side) and with the assistant positioned opposite

Patient positioning

- The patient should undergo a spinal anesthetic or a peripheral nerve or ankle block, which can offer pain relief during and after surgery
- A high thigh tourniquet should be applied and the patient positioned in the lateral decubitius position. The pelvis should be stabilized with a bolster on either side of it. The contralateral knee is flexed to 90°. Softs pads need to be applied to prevent possible pressure sores (**Figure 22.1**)
- One dose of antibiotic prophylaxis should be administered prior to exsanguination of the limb and inflation of the tourniquet to 300 mmHg

Surgical technique

Exposure

- This depends on the clinical picture and the type of lesion. Numerous techniques for tendon repair have been described

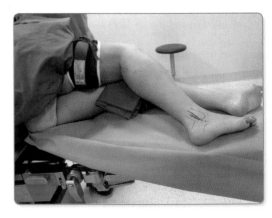

Figure 22.1 Patient positioning: lateral decubitus stabilized with lateral pad, tourniquet at the thigh.

Tendon repair

- This may be performed for isolated peroneus brevis tears, isolated peroneus longus tears, or both
- A slightly curved, 8–10 cm long longitudinal incision is made starting posterior to the lateral malleolus and directed towards the tip of the fifth metatarsal over the course of the peroneal tendons (**Figure 22.2**)
- The sural nerve must be identified and retracted, particularly if a more distal rupture is being treated because the nerve crosses the tendons distally
- The retinaculum is assessed for redundancy or elevation from the lateral surface of the fibula
- Once the retinaculum is opened longitudinally, leave a 4 mm cuff of tissue anteriorly so that the repair can be performed without constriction of the tendons (**Figure 22.3**)
- Deep to the retinaculum, fibrous and loose fragmented tissue is resected (**Figure 22.4**)
- Small longitudinal tears that result in splaying with minimal degeneration (**Figure 22.5**) or fraying are repaired with tubularization of the tendon using a running 4-0 absorbable suture (**Figure 22.6**)
- If the viable portion of the tendon comprises greater than 50% of the tendon diameter (**Figure 22.7**), the degenerated portion should be completely excised and the viable tendon repaired longitudinally with a running 4-0 absorbable suture (**Figure 22.8**)

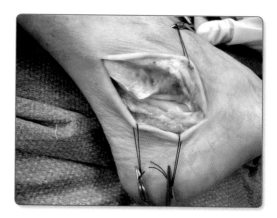

Figure 22.3 Incision of the peroneal sheath.

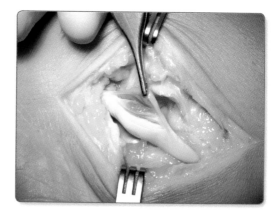

Figure 22.4 Resection of loose fragment of tendon lesion.

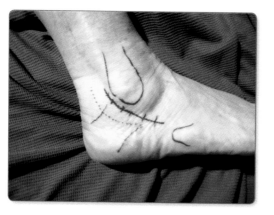

Figure 22.2 Skin incision over the course of the peroneal tendons.

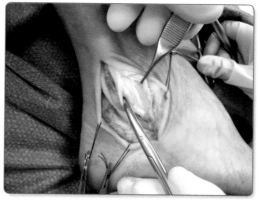

Figure 22.5 Longitudinal lesion of peroneus brevis tendon (stage II).

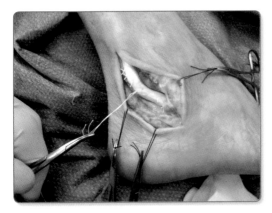

Figure 22.6 Tubularization of the tendon lesion.

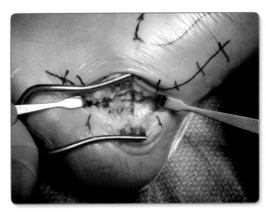

Figure 22.9 Additional posterior incision for calcaneal osteotomy.

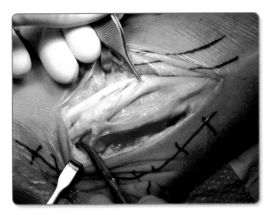

Figure 22.7 Wide lesion of peroneus brevis tendon.

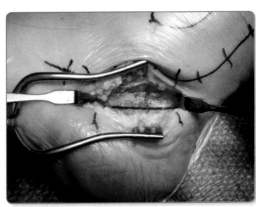

Figure 22.10 Oblique osteotomy of the calcaneum.

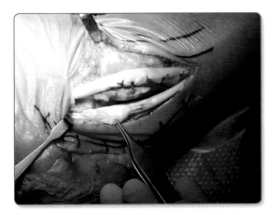

Figure 22.8 Same lesion after the repair.

- Tubularizing the tendon re-establishes a smooth tendon. If the viable portion of the tendon is less than 50% of the cross-sectional area, the degenerated portion is debrided and a proximal and distal tenodesis of the brevis tendon to the longus tendon can be performed with a 2–0 absorbable suture
- An absorbable suture is used to avoid persistent irritation within the tendon sheath. To avoid fibular impingement, the proximal tenodesis should be placed at least 3–4 cm above the tip of the lateral malleolus, and the distal tenodesis should be placed at least 5–6 cm below the tip of the lateral malleolus
- The superior peroneal retinaculum is repaired either by direct suture or, if it is totally

incompetent, by advancing the posterior flap and securing it through a series of drill holes in the posterolateral fibula

Tendon repair: tears of both the peroneus longus and brevis

- As with isolated tears of the peroneus brevis and longus, the type of rupture and the amount of tendon degeneration must be assessed intraoperatively
- If both tendons are grossly intact, they are repaired in a standard manner by excising the longitudinal tear and tubularizing the remaining tendon with a running absorbable 4-0 suture
- If one tendon is completely torn and irreparable, but the other tendon is considered functional (**Figure 22.11**), a tenodesis is carried out proximally using musculotendinous tissue and any healthy tendon distal to the muscle (**Figure 22.12**)
- The decision to perform a tenodesis is also based on the state of the muscle and the amount of excursion (the difference between the maximum shortening and maximum lengthening of the muscle) it has
- If the both tendons are nonfunctional, a tendon graft or tendon transfer of the flexor digitorum longus (FDL) to the peroneus brevis is recommended
- If no excursion of the proximal muscle is evident, an FDL transfer is the procedure of choice
- If there is adequate tendon excursion, an allograft tendon reconstruction is the procedure of choice
- Either procedure can be performed in one or two stages, depending on the state of the tendon bed
- After excision of the degenerated tendon, the tendon bed is assessed for scarring
- If minimal or no scarring is present, the procedure of choice can be performed in the same setting
- If scarring is present, the surgery must be staged. This first stage re-establishes a synovial cavity with the use of a silicone rod

Tendon repair: silicone rod technique

- A longitudinal incision is made 5 cm proximal and 6 cm distal to the tip of the

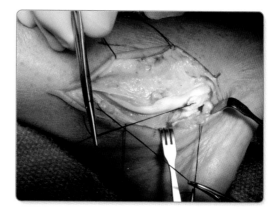

Figure 22.11 Complete transversal lesion of peroneus longus tendon.

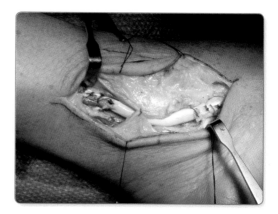

Figure 22.12 Tenodesis of the torn peroneus longus to peroneus brevis.

fibula over the course of the peroneal tendons
- The excursion and function of the tendons is checked. If some excursion of the musculotendinous unit is present, an allograft tendon reconstruction is planned
- If muscle fibrosis prevents excursion of the tendon, an FDL transfer is planned
- The degenerated tendon is excised, leavings mall stumps proximally and distally
- After excision of the scarred tendons, the tendon bed is assessed for scarring
- If scarring is present, a silicone rod is inserted and attached distally to the remaining stump of the peroneus brevis tendon; the proximal end is left free to allow some motion of the rod. The incision is closed and early motion is allowed

- The procedure of choice is performed 6 weeks later once there is a synovial cavity

Tendon repair: hamstring allograft reconstruction

- As a single-stage procedure, the allograft reconstruction is relatively straightforward
- After excision of the degenerated tendon, a hamstring allograft is attached to the proximal muscle and tendon using 2-0 FiberWire suture
- If there is a substantial brevis stump, the allograft is sutured into the distal tendon; however, a loss of viable tendon may necessitate insertion into the base of the fifth metatarsal with suture anchors
- For the second stage of a hamstring allograft reconstruction the approach is different from that for a primary reconstruction
- Two incisions are made; the proximal incision exposes only the rod–tendon junction, and the distal incision exposes only the attachment site distally
- This technique avoids reopening the entire wound and preserves the synovial cavity created by the silicone rod
- Once the proximal silicone stump is exposed, the hamstring allograft is attached to the myotendinous junction, and the distal end is attached to the free end of the silicone rod
- The distal incision is made and, as the rod is removed through the distal wound, the distal tendon is drawn into the synovial cavity and down to the fifth metatarsal base
- The tendon is then attached distally to the base of the fifth metatarsal with a suture anchor or to the distal brevis stump
- It is important to apply adequate tension to the allograft

Tendon repair: flexor digitorum longus transfer to the peroneus brevis

- In a single-stage procedure, the FDL tendon is harvested after excision of the degenerated peroneal tendon
- On the medial side, a double approach is used to expose the FDL
- A small 1 or 2 cm incision is made just below the medial portion of the abductor hallucis muscle on the medial plantar aspect of the midfoot; the FDL is identified at the master knot of Henry and followed distally

- The tendon is transected as distally as possible to maintain length
- A tenodesis of the FDL to the flexor hallucis longus before transaction of the FDL is not necessary
- The tendon is tagged with a Kessler-type suture. A second smaller incision is made proximal and posterior to the medial malleolus; the sheath over the FDL is opened and the tendon is pulled proximally
- The tendon is then rerouted across the deep compartment, posterior to the neurovascular bundle and anterior to the Achilles tendon, to the lateral fibula, and into the incision
- The tendon is routed along the peroneal brevis tendon bed and attached to the base of the fifth metatarsal with the foot in maximal eversion
- In a two-stage procedure, a small incision is made in the proximal and distal aspects of the lateral wound, identical to that in the staged allograft procedure
- After retrieval of the tendon to the posterior aspect of the medial malleolus, the tendon is routed laterally, posterior to the neurovascular bundle and anterior to the Achilles tendon
- The tendon is introduced into the proximal lateral incision and tied to the silicone rod, which is then removed through the distal incision, thereby transferring the FDL tendon into the synovial cavity
- The rod is then removed from its attachment to the FDL, and the tendon is attached to the base of the fifth metatarsal via suture anchors while the foot is held in maximal eversion

Additional procedures

- If there is a varus deformity of the hindfoot a Dwyer's osteotomy of the calcaneus may be indicated
- Usually, this is performed through an additional oblique incision parallel to the previous one and 2.5–3 cm posteriorly (**Figure 22.9**)
- The subcutaneous tissue is divided, protecting the sural nerve in the anterior flap. The lateral aspect of the calcaneus in isolated and two Hohmann retractors are placed in the dorsal and plantar edges of the os calcis
- A cuneiform resection is made with an oscillating saw perpendicular to the longitudinal axis of the calcaneus

- The amount resected is about 10–15 mm depending on the deformity (**Figure 22.10**); the medial calcaneal cortex should be scored and fractured during the reduction
- The osteotomized surfaces are compressed together and held with two 2.5 mm Kirschner (K)-wires or staples
- If there is lateral instability of the ankle, nsurgical stabilization should be considered: usually, the Bromstrom–Gould technique is performed

Possible perioperative complications

- Poor quality of the suture: check the quality of the suture in flexion and inversion

Closure

- The retinaculum and fat should be repaired with absorbable sutures, the skin closed in the standard fashion, and a simple dressing placed
- There is no need to place a wound drain
- The foot is immobilized in a removable boot for 4 weeks, followed by a removable stirrup splint for another 4 weeks

Postoperative management

Postoperative regimen

- Prescribed medications should include analgesics, nonsteroidal anti-inflammatory drugs, and thromboembolic prevention (which is given for 30 days)
- Active range of motion is initiated at 3 weeks
- At 4 weeks, full weight bearing begins
- At 8 weeks, patients begin a supervised physiotherapy program to emphasize strengthening and proprioception

Outpatient follow-up

- Complications are subdivided into minor andmajor complications:
  - Minor complications include transient sural neuritis, tendonitis symptoms, and asymptomatic peroneal subluxation
  - Maior complications include hematoma, wound dehiscence, nonresolution, or recurrence of tendonitis, and an unstable ankle

Further reading

Demetracopoulos CA, Vineyard JC, Kiesau CD, et al. Long-term results of debridement and primary repair of peroneal tendon tears. Foot Ankle Int 2014 ;35:252–257.

Sobel M, Geppert MJ, Olson EJ, et al. The dynamics of peroneus brevis tendon splits: a proposed mechanism, technique of diagnosis, and classification of injury. Foot Ankle 1992; 13:413–422.

Stamatis ED, Karaoglanis GC. Salvage options for peroneal tendon ruptures. Foot Ankle Clin 2014; 19:87–95.

Stockton KG, Brodsky JW. Peroneus longus tears associated with pathology of the os peroneum. Foot Ankle Int 2014; 35:346–352.

23 Posterior tibialis tendon reconstruction

Indications

Reconstruction of the posterior tibialis tendon (PTT) is indicated in PTT dysfunction (PTTD) only if hindfoot deformity is not present (as this necessitates osteotomy or arthrodesis).

- Many PTTD staging systems have been developed; however the most widely used is the Johnson and Strom classification, later modified by Myerson (**Table 23.1**). Surgical treatment is advised for stages II and above
- In the early stages of PTTD, the flatfoot deformity is correctable and the heel is supple. This indicates that reconstruction of the PTT may be effective
- Stage II PTT insufficiency in young patients represents the ideal indication for the PTT reconstruction with flexor digitorum longus (FDL) transfer and lateral column lengthening combined with a medializing calcaneal osteotomy
- Although less common than the chronic degenerative scenario, acute PTTD is usually caused by ankle trauma in abduction–pronation during sporting activities
- Traumatic lacerations of the PTT may be associated with an ankle fracture and dislocation

- The degenerative disease process of the PTT may develop in diabetes mellitus, hypertension, rheumatoid arthritis, obesity, and steroid overuse
- Chronic degeneration can lead to an acute tendon rupture
- In chronic cases the damage to the PTT is frequently caused by 'overuse injuries' associated with a twisting motion, as seen in sports like tennis, basketball, and soccer
- If conservative treatment is ineffective, surgery should be considered promptly as the PTT is an important dynamic stabilizer and the most powerful inverter of the foot
- Correct diagnosis of PTTD is vital. Differential diagnoses include plantar fasciitis, tendinosis, and subtalar and talonavicular synovitis (Premkumar, 2002)

Risk factors

- The main risk factors for a PTTD are:
  - Hyperpronation of the foot during sports activities
  - Flatfoot deformity
  - Flexible pes planovalgus
- The adult acquired flatfoot may be caused by:
  - Neuropathic (Charcot) foot, secondary to diabetes, leprosy, or peripheral neuropathy

Table 23.1 Modified Johnson and Strom classification for posterior tibialis tendon dysfunction

	Stage I	Stage II	Stage III	Stage IV
Tendon condition	Mild inflammatory state	Elongation of the tendon	Elongation of the tendon	Marked degeneration of the tendon
Pain	Pain	Pain	Pain	Valgus deformity of the ankle joint
Deformity	No structural deformity	Flexible flatfoot deformity	Fixed flatfoot deformity	Arthritis of the ankle
Weakness	Mild	Forefoot abduction when weight bearing	Forefoot abduction when weight bearing	Forefoot abduction when weight bearing
Single heel-rise test	Complete single heel rise with inversion of the heel	No or limited inversion of hindfoot in single heel rise	Inability to perform the test	Inability to perform the test

- Degenerative changes of the ankle, secondary to primary or post-traumatic osteoarthritis
- Loss of the supporting structures of the medial longitudinal arch, for example a tear of the spring (calcaneonavicular) ligament or rupture of the anterior tibialis tendon
- Risk of rupture of the PTT is also determined by its acute angulation
- As the PTT passes posterior to the medial malleolus, this zone of hypovascularity distal to the medial malleolus may contribute to the development of PTT degeneration and failure

Contraindications

- A complete chronic rupture of the PTT requires arthrodesis: tendon reconstruction and a calcaneal osteotomy is not effective

Preoperative assessment

Clinical assessment

Clinical presentation

- In its early stages, discomfort is perceived along the medial malleolus and arch of the foot
- As the process intensifies, the hindfoot deformity develops and pain shifts on the lateral side of the ankle, as the fibula impinges on the calcaneus

Physical examination

- A comparative evaluation of both ankles should be performed
- Lower leg and hindfoot alignment must be investigated with the patient standing: genu valgum may accentuate the flatfoot deformity
- Stability and proprioceptive control of the ankle may be examined by asking the patient to stand on one leg
- PTTD is highly suggested if a patient cannot perform a single leg heel rise
- The integrity of the tendon and the point of maximum tenderness should be evaluated, especially by inspecting for swelling behind the medial malleolus (**Figure 23.1**)
- Active subtalar inversion and eversion provokes pain
- A thorough ankle examination should be performed, including paying particular attention to the Achilles tendon
- Increased valgus angulation of the heel gradually causes a lateral move of the

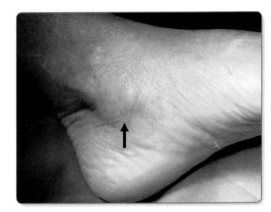

Figure 23.1 Tibialis posterior swelling evident under the medial malleolus.

Achilles tendon to the axis of the subtalar joint, and the gastrocnemius muscle group shortens

- The foot may change shape over time. The heel tilts into valgus, while the longitudinal arch gradually collapses, leading to the development of a hindfoot valgus
- The strength of the PTT can be assessed asking the patient to bring the foot into an inverted and plantarflexed position, while the clinician exerts counter resistance
- Valgus angulation of the hindfoot and abduction of the forefoot are noticeable if the foot is seen from behind. When looking at the heel from the back of the patient, the clinician usually sees only the fifth toe and half of the fourth one. According to the 'too many toes' sign, the lesser toes can be seen on the affected side with hindfoot valgus and forefoot abduction in presence of a chronic degeneration of the PTT (Trnka, 2004)
- When the patient stands on tiptoes, the heel usually swings in a varus direction. In PTTD, standing on tiptoes is very difficult and the heels remain in valgus
- Navicular drop test is performed to assess the height of the navicular tuberosity. The amount of excursion is measured between the stance and the neutral positions (Brody, 1982). Values greater than 10 mm can be considered abnormal (Loudon, 1996)
- Further mechanical information may be evaluated with the baropodometric examination. This accurately assesses loads through the feet on standing and walking.

It is especially useful in congenital hindfoot deformity and following an acute traumatic event, as the patient may modify the loads for antalgic reasons
- The physician may perform this examination before and after surgery to assess the outcomes after surgical treatment

Imaging assessment

Ultrasonography

- Because of its superficial location, PTT is particularly suitable for early ultrasonography
- The examination is performed with the patient in a prone oblique position and the ankle slightly elevated. Color and power Doppler ultrasonography may be used to assess tendon and paratendinous areas
- A healthy PTT usually shows a diameter between 4 and 6 mm and appears hyperechoic (Trnka, 2004)
- The most important ultrasonography criteria are:
  - Measurement of the diameter of both the PTT and FDL tendons
  - The signal intensity of the tendons
  - The echogenicity of the tendons
  - The presence of flow within the tendons on color and power Doppler imaging
  - The presence of fluid and hypoechoic tissue in the peritendon area (Premkumar, 2002)
- In chronic degenerative PTTD, the tendon may appear thickened, more or less fusiform and hypoechoic
- Gradually, microfractures may develop as longitudinal fissures, and the tendon eventually loses its normal mechanical characteristics
- For a correct evaluation, the size of the PPT should be compared to that of the flexor of the adjacent toes (Lhoste-Trouilloud, 2012)
- Sonographic parameters for a PTT synovitis are:
  - Inflammatory fluids surrounding the tendon
  - An irregular contour
  - Heterogeneous echogenicity

Magnetic resonance imaging (MRI)

- MRI is useful for detecting tendonitis and assessing tendon tears
- MRI is usually performed in the neutral position, obtaining sagittal images along the plane of the PTT and axial images perpendicular to that plane

- The most common findings are contrast enhancement and abnormal signal intensity of the tendon (Premkumar, 2002)
- Currently, MRI is the best method for assessing tendon ruptures. Size, shape, and internal signal are best seen on axial sections

Radiographs

- Radiographs help the surgeon to evaluate the hindfoot alignment, especially if a flatfoot deformity is present
- It is important to assess the ankle alignment in all the three planes on weight-bearing radiographs. Useful parameters include:
  - The ankle between the talus and first metatarsal
  - The talonavicular uncoverage angle
  - The arch height at the medial cuneiform (Arangio, 2006)

Computed tomography (CT)

- CT may be helpful not only for its accuracy, but also because arthritis at the back of the foot has similar symptoms to PTTD
- In the delineation of tendon calcification and retinacular avulsion of bone, CT is superior to MRI; nevertheless, CT and MRI are almost of equal value for detecting PTT abnormalities

Timing for surgery

- Surgery takes place preferably if there is no progressive swelling and after conservative treatment has failed

Surgical preparation

Special surgical considerations

- A calcaneal osteotomy is indicated in case of hindfoot malalignment, otherwise only PTT reconstruction is performed
- The calcaneal osteotomy modifies the valgus angulation by medializing the calcaneal axis and therefore correcting the mechanical axis of the lower limb. In turn, this slightly redirects the pull of the gastrocnemius muscle group, increasing the varus pull on the hindfoot
- A valgus hindfoot requires a medial slide calcaneal osteotomy and FDL transfer for reconstruction of the PTT. Additional techniques include lateral column lengthening and spring ligament reconstruction

Surgical equipment

- Needle holder
- Sutures
- Scalpels, blades no. 11 and 21
- Forceps: toothed tissue forceps, Adson's tissue forceps, Kocher's, Kelly's, and mosquito forceps
- Scissors
- Oscillating saw
- Luer bone rongeur
- Farabeuf retractors
- Mini Hohmann bone elevators
- Bone curettes
- Mallet
- Osteotome
- Drill equipment: hand drill, drill guide, and drill bits
- Kirschner wires
- Screws
- Screwdriver

Equipment positioning

- The surgical equipment is positioned near the surgeon, on the same side of the ankle to be operated on

Patient positioning

- The patient is positioned supine
- A tourniquet is placed on the thigh
- At the appropriate time, the foot, ankle, and leg are exanguinated and the tourniquet is inflated

Further preparation

- The patient receives a single dose of intravenous antibiotics
- Local anesthesia is infiltrated

Surgical technique

Medial calcaneal osteotomy

- A 4 cm oblique incision is made over the lateral aspect of the calcaneal tuberosity, behind the lateral malleolus, parallel to the peroneal sheath, and posterior to the sural nerve
- After reflection of the periosteum, a transverse calcaneal osteotomy is performed using an oscillating saw and completed with an osteotome
- The tuberosity fragment is medially translated about 1 cm and fixed by a cannulated cancellous lag screw

Transfer of flexor digitorum longus (PTT reconstruction)

- A medial incision is performed along the medial column of the foot (**Figure 23.2**). It starts from the medial malleolus and then passes beyond the navicular tuberosity, following the inferior border of the first metatarsal
- The sheath of the PTT is opened; the tendon is inspected (**Figures 23.3** and **23.4**)
- The PTT is repaired with absorbable stitches (**Figure 23.5**)
- The FDL sheath is identified and opened, just below the medial malleolus (**Figure 23.6**) to augment the PTT

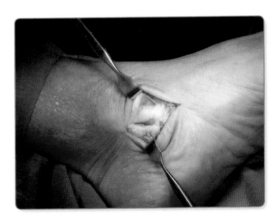

Figure 23.2 Skin incision: tourniquet inflated.

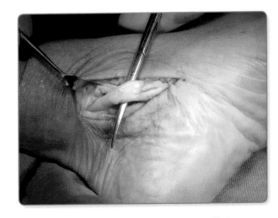

Figure 23.3 Tendon degeneration and partial lesion.

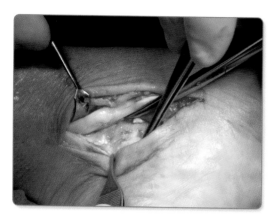

Figure 23.4 Inflamed paratenon.

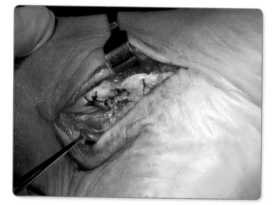

Figure 23.5 Tendon repaired with absorbable stitches.

- After the identification of the flexor hallucis longus, a distal tenodesis of both flexor hallucis longus and FDL can be performed, and the FDL is cut. This tenodesis may also be unnecessary, since several connections exist between the two tendons
- The FDL constitutes only the 30% of the PTT strength, so its transfer needs to be associated with the hindfoot medialization, in order to reduce the antagonistic forces in case of hindfoot malalignment
- After a dissection of the periosteum, a dorsal to plantar drill hole is made through the navicular tuberosity
- The FDL is passed through and sutured together with the PTT in the deep periosteum (Schuh, 2013) (**Figure 23.7**)
- To avoid overstretching, the optimal tension of the FDL should be set halfway between complete relaxation and maximum tension
- An intradermal suture is performed (**Figure 23.8**)
- The foot rests in a slight equinovarus position (Trnka, 2004)

Lengthening of the lateral column

- If a pes planovalgus deformity has developed, the lateral column of the foot shortens over time. For this reason, it should be lengthened to restore the medial longitudinal arch

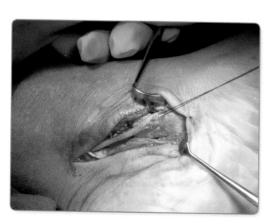

Figure 23.6 Flexor digitorum longus is detached distally and prepared for the augmentation.

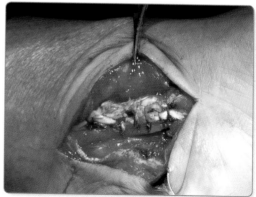

Figure 23.7 The flexor digitorum longus is sutured to the posterior tibialis tendon until its insertion site.

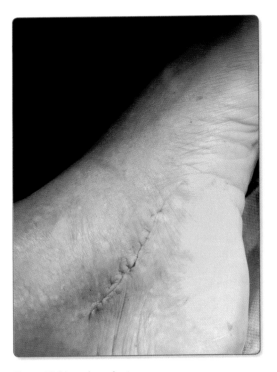

Figure 23.8 Intradermal sutures.

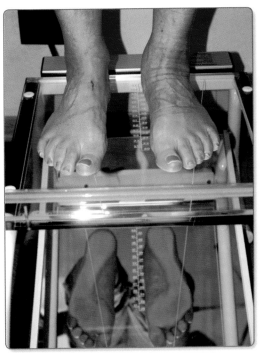

Figure 23.9 Standing evaluation 8 months later: the patient is still a runner after 10 years.

Possible perioperative complications

- It is important not to damage the closest neurovascular structures, such as the tibialis posterior artery and the tibialis posterior nerve

Closure

- After thorough irrigation with 0.9% saline, the skin incisions are sutured and Steri-Strips are applied
- A pneumatic ankle brace or a light cast is applied, keeping the ankle in slight dorsal flexion and eversion
- An elastic bandage is always applied over the skin to avoid distal edema

Postoperative management

Postoperative regimen

- Weight bearing is highly discouraged for the first 3–4 postoperative weeks. During the first 2 weeks, the patient is asked first to wear a plaster splint, and then a non weight-bearing cast until complete weight bearing is reached from 8–10 weeks
- First week post-operatively: Ice, elevation of the foot, medications such as pain relievers, nonsteroidal anti-inflammatory drugs, and thrombosis and pulmonary embolism prevention are used
- 2 weeks postoperatively: radiographs are taken
- 6 weeks postoperatively: Physical therapy may be started, for active motion and strength recovery
- 1 month postoperatively: A soft bandage and orthotics may be helpful for a gradual recovery
- 3 months postoperatively: Radiographs and a clinical evaluation (**Figure 23.9**) are undertaken

Early-phase postoperative complications

- Wound breakdown
- Infection
- Bleeding
- Nerve injury
- Instability or recurrence
- Complex regional pain syndrome

Outpatient follow-up

- Patients are assessed as described above and then at 6-monthly intervals for 2 years, being discharged at that stage

- Further examinations will be necessary only if symptoms develop again or if a new trauma occurs

Further reading

Arangio GA, Wasser T, Rogman A. Radiographic comparison of standing medial cuneiform arch height in adults with and without acquired flatfoot deformity. Foot Ankle Int 2006; 27:636–638.

Brody TM. Techniques in the evaluation and treatment of the injured runner. Orthop Clin North Am 1982; 13:541–558.

Gluck GS, Heckman DS, Parekh SG. Tendon disorders of the foot and ankle, part 3: the posterior tibial tendon. Am J Sports Med 2010; 38:2133–2144.

Kohls-Gatzoulis J, Angel JC, Singh D, et al. Tibialis posterior dysfunction: a common and treatable cause of adult acquired flatfoot. BMJ 2004; 329:1328–1333.

Lhoste-Trouilloud A. The tibialis posterior tendon. J Ultrasound 2012; 15:2–6.

Loudon JK, Jenkins W, Loudon KL. The relationship between static posture and ACL injury in female athletes. J Orthop Sports Phys Ther 1996; 24:91–97.

Premkumar A, Perry MB, Dwyer AJ, et al. Sonography and MR imaging of posterior tibial tendinopathy. AJR Am J Roentgenol 2002; 178:223–232.

Schuh R, Gruber F, Wanivenhaus A, et al. Flexor digitorum longus transfer and medial displacement calcaneal osteotomy for the treatment of stage II posterior tibial tendon dysfunction: kinematic and functional results of fifty one feet. Int Orthop 2013; 37:1815–1820.

Trnka HJ. Dysfunction of the tendon of tibialis posterior. J Bone Joint Surg Br 2004; 86:939–946.

Management of posterior tibialis tendon dislocation

Indications

- Isolated traumatic dislocations are rare. In these cases, acute trauma occurs frequently combined with an inversion and dorsiflexion or plantarflexion of the ankle
- The exact diagnosis is often delayed due to previous treatments for ankle sprains, tendonitis, or subtalar dislocation (Mitchell, 2011). For this reason, the average time to diagnosis may be up to 9 months (Ouzanian, 1992)
- Differential diagnosis includes:
  - Posterior tibialis tendon (PTT) rupture
  - Sprain of the deltoid ligament
  - Fracture of the posteromedial process of the talus
  - Fracture of the navicular tuberosity
- An exact diagnosis is fundamental for fast and effective treatment, in order to avoid subsequent hindfoot instability and flattening of the medial longitudinal arch (Gambardella, 2014)
- Conservative treatment for a PTT dislocation is usually unsuccessful, with persistent pain and swelling. However, it may be effective if the PTT is relatively anatomically positioned and if ankle immobilization can be started early

Risk factors

- The most common mechanism of injury is a traumatic event
- The foot is inverted and dorsiflexed, with a sudden and violent contraction of the PTT
- An example of a nontraumatic mechanism of injury is lifting from a squatting position without raising the heels
- A shallow PTT groove is considered a predisposing factor for tendon dislocation (Soler, 1986)
- A tear or an avulsion of the flexor retinaculum, a lax retinaculum, chronic repetitive trauma, and a previous medial malleolar fracture that has left structural disorders may all also lead to a PTT dislocation (Gambardella, 2014)
- Multiple steroid injections and tarsal tunnel release are further examples of predisposing factors for PTT dislocation (Ouzanian, 1992; Langan, 1980)

Preoperative assessment

Clinical assessment

Clinical presentation

- The patient may complain of medial ankle pain, refractory to conservative treatment. It can develop suddenly during sport or daily activities
- Pain may be associated with swelling over the medial malleolus and possible posterior ecchymosis
- A recurrent feeling of snapping at the medial ankle is usually present
- Loss of PTT function gradually causes an incorrect posture and walking stance, leading to development of a flatfoot deformity

Physical examination

- The diagnosis of this kind of injury is often delayed and not easily assessed: if the tendon has subluxed anteriorly to the malleolus and does not repeatedly dislocate, the evaluation may be difficult (Miki, 1998)
- A comparative assessment of both ankles is always necessary, including a check of stability and proprioceptive control
- The integrity of the tendon and the point of maximum tenderness should be evaluated, especially inspecting for swelling behind the medial malleolus (**Figure 24.1**)
- The dislocated tendon usually reduces with tibiotalar plantarflexion and redislocates with dorsiflexion
- Whereas the functional assessment of the tibiotarsal joint may be normal, the demonstration of tendon dislocation may

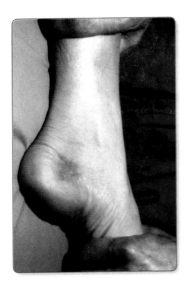

Figure 24.1
Posterior tibialis tendon dislocated over the medial malleolus: an acute lesion.

be evoked with resisted plantarflexion and inversion of the foot. The clinician may frequently check the tendon dislocation anterior to the medial malleolus, performing an opposed contraction of the tibialis posterior muscle. During this test the patient may feel a painful 'click'
- Pain and swelling are usually located in the retromalleolar area, followed by tenderness anterior to the medial malleolus when the swelling has passed away
- The strength of the PTT can be assessed by asking the patient to bring the foot into an inverted and plantarflexed position, while the clinician exerts counterresistance. Strength tests are frequently normal

Imaging assessment

Ultrasonography
- Ultrasonography is particularly useful for early evaluation of the PTT, because of the superficial location of the tendon
- The examination is performed with the patient in a prone oblique position and the ankle slightly elevated. Color and power Doppler imaging may be used to assess the tendon and paratendon areas.
- A healthy PTT usually shows a diameter between 4 and 6 mm and appears hyperechoic (Trnka, 2004)
- The most important criteria are:
  - Measurement of the diameter of both the PTT and flexor digitorum longus tendons

- The signal intensity of the tendons
- The echogenicity of the tendons
- The presence of flow within the tendons on color and power Doppler imaging
- The presence of fluid and hypoechoic tissue in the peritendon area (Premkumar, 2002)
- The pathognomonic sign of PTT dislocation is a displacement of the tendon anteriorly to the medial malleolus, associated with soft tissue inflammatory signs

Magnetic resonance imaging (MRI)
- According to some authors, MRI is the gold standard for radiologic investigation in cases of PTT dislocation (Mitchell, 2011)
- MRI is usually performed in the neutral position, obtaining sagittal images along the plane of the PTT and axial images perpendicular to that plane
- The size, shape, and internal signal of the PTT are best seen on axial sections
- MRI generally shows the displaced PTT, a raised or torn flexor retinaculum and/or a hypoplastic retromalleolar groove (Gambardella, 2014)

Radiographs
- Radiographs are of minimal use in the direct diagnosis of PTT dislocation. They may reveal a medial malleolus fracture

Computed tomography (CT)
- CT may be helpful for detecting the dislocation, although MRI remains the gold standard

Timing for surgery
- Surgery takes place in the acute setting
- In cases of a swollen ankle, surgery takes place when the swelling has largely decreased

Surgical preparation
Special surgical considerations
- The PTT is strongly held in the retromalleolar groove by the flexor retinaculum and a fibro-osseous tunnel. The PTT dislocation is usually caused by a tear of these structures
- The flexor digitorum longus, the flexor hallucis longus, and the posterior tibial neurovascular bundle lie deeper than the PTT. For this reason they are rarely involved in the dislocation

Surgical equipment

- Needle holder
- Sutures
- Scalpels, blades no. 11 and 21
- Forceps: toothed tissue forceps, Adson's tissue forceps, Kocher's, Kelly's, and mosquito forceps
- Scissors
- Farabeuf retractors
- Mini Hohmann bone elevators
- Bone curettes

Equipment positioning

- The surgical equipment is positioned near the surgeon, on the same side of the ankle to be operated on

Patient positioning

- The patient is placed supine
- A tourniquet is positioned on the thigh
- At the appropriate time, the foot, ankle, and leg are exsanguinated and the tourniquet is inflated

Further preparation

- The patient receives a single dose of intravenous antibiotics preoperatively
- Local anesthesia is infiltrated

Surgical technique

Tissue dissection

- A curvilinear incision is made along the posterior aspect of the medial malleolus
- The thick retinaculum is exposed: proximal detachment from the medial malleolus is clearly evident (**Figure 24.2**)
- The PTT integrity is evaluated (**Figure 24.3**)
- The PTT is released from the scar tissue in chronic cases

Retinaculum repair

- The retinaculum is repaired by applying 2-0 absorbable stitches (**Figure 24.4**)
- Before closure, the surgeon evaluates the mobility and stability of the PTT: it is particularly important to assess the sliding of the tendon into the fibro-osseous groove beneath the retinaculum

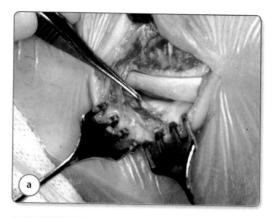
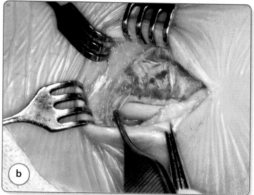

Figure 24.2 After a longitudinal skin incision has been made below the medial malleolus (a), the tendon retinaculum is exposed (b).

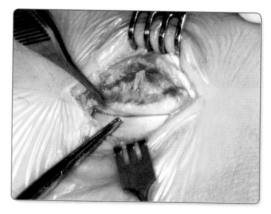

Figure 24.3 Retinaculum disruption: the posterior tibialis tendon is not damaged.

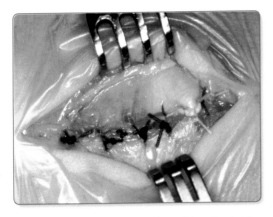

Figure 24.4 Suture of the retinaculum with reabsorbable stitches.

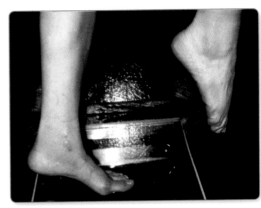

Figure 24.5 Joint function restored few months later.

Possible perioperative complications

- It is important not to damage the closest neurovascular structures, such as the tibialis posterior artery and the tibialis posterior nerve
- Immediately beneath the PTT, the flexor digitorum longus tendon should be isolated and left untouched

Closure

- After thorough irrigation with 0.9% saline, the skin incisions are sutured and Steri-Strips are applied
- An elastic bandage is applied to avoid distal edema
- A plaster boot is applied to stabilize the ankle joint

Postoperative management

Postoperative regimen

- Weight bearing is discouraged for the first 3–4 postoperative weeks
- During the first month, the patient is asked to wear a plaster boot in order to let the tissues heal and to avoid a new dislocation until complete weight bearing is reached within 6 weeks

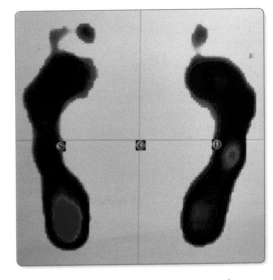

Figure 24.6 Baropodometric evaluation 25 years later.

- The patient usually is able to resume sports activities at 12 weeks postoperatively (**Figures 24.5–24.7**)

Early-phase postoperative complications

- Wound breakdown
- Infection
- Bleeding
- Nerve injury
- Instability or recurrence
- Complex regional pain syndrome

Outpatient follow-up

- Patients are assessed at 6-monthly intervals for 2 years and then discharged at that stage
- Further examinations will be necessary only if symptoms develop again or if a new trauma occurs

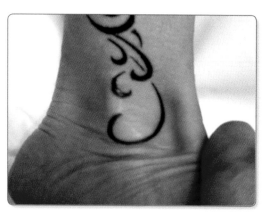

Figure 24.7 Posterior tibialis tendon stability 25 years later.

Further reading

Canata GL. Lussazione traumatica del tibiale posteriore. Sports Traumatol 1987; 9:307–309.

Gambardella GV, Donegan R, Caminear DS. Isolated dislocation of the posterior tibial tendon in an amateur snowboarder: a case report. J Foot Ankle Surg 2014; 53:203–207.

Goucher NR, Coughlin MJ, Kristensen RM. Dislocation of the posterior tibial tendon: a literature review and presentation of two cases. Iowa Orthop J 2006; 26:122–126.

Langan P, Weiss CA. Subluxation of the tibialis posterior, a complication of tarsal tunnel decompression: a case report. Clin Orthop Relat Res 1980; 146:226–227.

Miki T, Kuzuoka K, Kotani H, Ikeda Y. Recurrent dislocation of tibialis posterior tendon. A report of two cases. Arch Orthop Trauma Surg 1998; 118:96–98.

Mitchell K, Mencia MM, Hoford R. Tibialis posterior tendon dislocation: a case report. Foot (Edinb) 1998; 118:96–98.

Ouzounian TJ, Myerson MS. Dislocation of the posterior tibial tendon. Foot Ankle 1992; 13:215–219.

Phisitkul P, Amendola N. Athletic injuries of the foot and the ankle. In: Parekh SG (ed.), Foot and ankle surgery. New Delhi: Jaypee Brothers Medical Publishers (P) Ltd, 2012: 409.

Premkumar A, Perry MB, Dwyer AJ, et al. Sonography and MR imaging of posterior tibial tendinopathy. Am J Roentgenol 2002; 178:223–232.

Soler RR, Gallart Castany FJ, Riba Ferret J, et al. Traumatic dislocation of the tibialis posterior tendon at the ankle level. J Trauma 1986; 26:1049–1052.

Trnka HJ. Dysfunction of the tendon of tibialis posterior. J Bone Joint Surg Br 2004; 86:939–946.

Surgical release of plantar fasciitis

Indications

Surgical release of the plantar fascia is indicated:

- When the patient has been suffering from continued unremitting pain for more than 6 months or longer, with failure of nonoperative treatment
- When the plantar fascia thickness is greater than 6 mm

Conservative measures

Conservative treatment of plantar fasciitis is successful in 90% of cases, usually reducing the symptoms within 9–12 months of onset. These measures include:

- Rest, activity modification, ice, and massage
- Oral analgesia and nonsteroidal anti-inflammatory drugs (NSAIDs):
  - NSAIDs have been shown to improve pain relief and disability in the interval between 2 and 6 months
  - In patients with seronegative disease, NSAIDs can produce a dramatic response, especially when combined with effective taping or strapping for managing plantar fasciitis
- Taping: There is no evidence on effect or benefit
- Steroid injections:
  - These are commonly used in the treatment of acute and chronic plantar fasciitis and have proven effect in the short term
  - Evidence suggests that they can cause fat pad atrophy and, very occasionally, may precipitate rupture of the plantar fascia
- Stretching of the calf muscles, Achilles tendon, and plantar fascia itself is an easily implementable treatment option:
  - In a prospective randomized controlled trial that compared these two approaches, researchers found that patients who stretched the plantar fascia showed a greater decrease in pain at its peak severity

and a decrease in pain with the first steps in the morning. Both groups experienced an overall decrease in pain

- Orthotics:
  - Night splints hold the foot in a neutral position, preventing contracture of the fascia during the sleep. This can particularly help to alleviate symptoms in the morning
  - Posterior-tension night splints maintain ankle dorsiflexion and toe extension, creating a constant mild stretch of the plantar fascia, allowing it to heal at a functional length
  - One Cochrane Review found limited evidence to support the use of night splints to treat patients with pain lasting more than 6 months. Patients treated with custom-made night splints improved, but patients treated with prefabricated night splints did not
- Heel inserts are a popular treatment adjunct and can be beneficial in relieving heel pain. Many types of shoe inserts have been used to manage plantar fasciitis:
  - One randomized controlled trial showed that magnet-embedded insoles were no more effective than placebo insoles in alleviating pain
  - Another study that compared custom orthotics and prefabricated shoe inserts (e.g. silicone heel pads, felt pads, rubber heel cups) combined with stretching found that the use of prefabricated insoles plus stretching was significantly more effective than custom orthotics plus stretching
- Botulinum toxin: Work looking into the effect of botulinum toxin injections to treat plantar fasciitis has shown apparently good effect, although this is still far from a mainstream treatment options
- Extracorporeal shockwave therapy (ESWT):
  - ESWT emerged in the early 1990s as an effective treatment of insertion tendinopathies. The mechanism of actions

of shockwaves is not fully understood and many theories have been proposed to explain it
- Proponents of ESWT believe that the shockwaves cause microdisruption of the thickened plantar fascia, resulting in an inflammatory response, revascularization, and recruitment of growth factors, and therefore a soft tissue reparative response
- ESWT should be regarded as an end-stage treatment for those patients who have failed conservative measures and are reluctant to have open surgery
- Shockwave therapy for the treatment of proximal plantar fasciopathy has a reported success rate ranging from 34% to 88%
- Several randomized, blinded, and controlled multicenter trials have demonstrated that shockwave therapy is more effective than placebo treatment
- Casting:
  - In one case series, investigators studied 32 patients with chronic heel pain who had not responded to multiple treatments
  - For 6 months, the patients wore well-padded fiberglass walking casts with the ankle in neutral to slight dorsiflexion and the toe plate in extension
  - At long-term follow-up, 25% of patients had complete resolution of their pain, and an additional 61% had some improvement
  - However, case series and other uncontrolled studies typically overestimate the benefits of treatment
- Protein-rich plasma:
  - At present there is a lack of good-quality evidence to support the efficacy of protein-rich plasma injections in the treatment of plantar fasciitis
  - The patient's own plasma is spun in a centrifuge and a specific fraction is then reinjected into the tender area
  - Blood and platelets, in particular, provide the richest source of these growth factors, storing and releasing them from their cytoplasmic α-granules
  - Platelets are one of the first cells to arrive at a site of injury, and can be activated by a large number of bioactive molecules, including thrombin, which itself has stimulatory properties in common with growth factors

- This and their capacity to release a multitude of growth factors means platelets are being explored as a delivery tool for growth factors and for their role in soft tissue healing
- The technique of deriving platelet-rich plasma preparations was developed in the 1990s for use in maxillofacial surgery, although its use has since spread to orthopaedic and plastic surgery, limb and myocardial ischemia, and ophthalmology
- Following the procedure, protocols vary, but the patient may use the limb normally, avoiding excessive or strenuous exercise and use for several weeks, be splinted, or undergo a formal rehabilitation program

Preoperative assessment
Clinical assessment
Basic signs of plantar fasciitis
- The patient will present with a history of pain located about the medial plantar aspect of the heel
- The onset of pain is often insidious
- Inferior heel pain occurs on weight bearing:
  - Pain may be throbbing, searing, or piercing, especially with the first few steps in the morning or after periods of inactivity
  - Once the patient starts walking, the pain tends to recede but then worsens with continued activity, such as prolonged walking or exercise, particularly on hard surfaces, often limiting daily activities
- Throughout the day, the patient may experience a burning sensation localized to the plantar aspect of the heel or extending anteriorly along the plantar fascia
- This burning sensation may proceed to frank pain after long periods of standing
- Palpation of the medial plantar calcaneal region will elicit a sharp, stabbing pain
- Passive ankle or first toe dorsiflexion can cause discomfort in the proximal plantar fascia; it can also assess tightness of the Achilles tendon
- Patients usually have tenderness around the medial calcaneal tuberosity at the plantar aponeurosis
- Walking barefoot, on toes, or up stairs may exacerbate the pain

- Patients may walk with their affected foot in an equinous position to avoid placing pressure on the painful heel

Further physical assessment

- Plantar fasciitis is more likely to occur in person who are obese, who spend most of the day on their feet, or who have limited ankle flexion
- Plantar fasciitis has also been shown to be associated with biomechanical abnormalities in the foot such as a tight Achilles tendon, pes cavus, and pes planus
- Excessive running also causes it

Differential diagnosis

- Neurologic:
  - Entrapment of the first branch of the lateral plantar nerve or the medial calcaneal nerve or abductor digiti minimi nerve
  - Tarsal tunnel syndrome
  - S1 radiculopathy
  - Neuropathies
  - Heel neuroma
  - Medial calcaneal neuritis
- Soft tissue:
  - Achilles tendonitis
  - Flabby heel syndrome with asteatosis of the calcaneal fat pad
  - Heel contusion
  - Plantar fascia rupture
  - Posterior tibial tendonitis
  - Retrocalcaneal or subcalcaneal bursitis
- Skeletal:
  - Calcaneal epiphysitis
  - Calcaneal stress fracture
  - Infection
  - Inflammatory arthropathies such as rheumatoid arthritis, Reiter's syndrome, ankylosing spondylitis, and psoriatic or gouty arthritis
  - Subtalar arthritis
  - Calcaneal periostitis
  - Osteomyelitis
- Miscellaneous:
  - Osteomalacia
  - Paget's disease
  - Sickle cell disease
  - Soft tissue or bone tumors
  - Vascular insufficiency
  - Fibromyalgia
  - Dermatologic conditions affecting the heel, such as fissures

Imaging assessment

- Imaging can aid in the diagnosis of plantar fasciitis. Although not routinely needed initially, imaging can be used to confirm recalcitrant plantar fasciitis or to rule out other heel pathology

Radiographs

- Plain radiography can identify bony lesions of the foot
- A bony spur may be present on a lateral projection, but this does not support the diagnosis of plantar fasciitis. Previous studies show that subcalcaneal spurs are also found in patients without plantar fasciitis (**Figure 25.1**)
- Radiographs may also show calcifications in the soft tissues around the heel or osteophytes on the anterior calcaneus

Ultrasonography

- This is inexpensive and useful in ruling out soft tissue pathology of the heel
- Findings that support the diagnosis of plantar fasciitis include a proximal plantar fascia thickness greater than 6 mm and areas of hypoechogenicity

Magnetic resonance imaging (MRI)

- MRI although expensive, is a valuable tool for assessing causes of recalcitrant heel pain
- MRI can show increased proximal plantar fascia thickening with increased signal intensity on T2-weighted and short tau inversion recovery images (**Figure 25.2**)
- MRI can identify other soft tissue lesions such as soft tissue tumors or the marrow edema

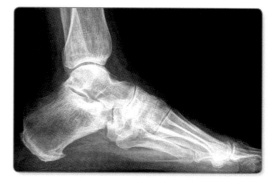

Figure 25.1 Lateral weight bearing radiograph showing bony plantar spur.

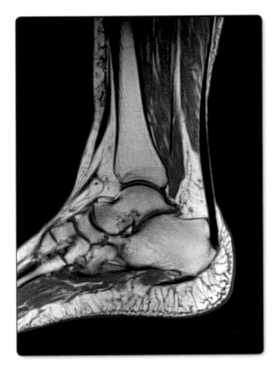

Figure 25.2 MRI of increased plantar fascia thickening.

associated with infection or MRI is used in an occult fracture is suspected

Electromyography
- This may be helpful if a neurogenic cause is suspected, such as S1 nerve root entrapment, tarsal tunnel syndrome, or entrapment of the lateral plantar nerve

Technetium bone scintigraphy
- This is positive in plantar fasciitis, with the maximum area of uptake at the point of maximum tenderness on the heel
- It also shows an area of increased uptake in the presence of an occult fracture

Timing for surgery
- The response to conservative measures is usually very good
- The proportion of patients requiring surgery is of the order of 1–2%
- Patients not responding to conservative measures after 6 months or longer may require surgery
- There is controversy as to which procedures are most likely to produce a good result, in part because of the limited scale of many published series

Surgical preparation

Surgical equipment
- No. 23 and no.15 blades
- Two retractors
- Adson's forceps
- Saw
- Luer rongeur or rasp
- Electrocautery
- Mayo scissors

Equipment positioning
- The surgical instruments face the surgeon on the opposite side of the table

Patient positioning
- The patient is placed in the supine position with external rotation of the limb and a soft support under the contralateral hip (**Figure 25.3**)
- A tourniquet is applied to the thigh

Further preparation
- One dose of antibiotic prophylaxis

Surgical technique

- Inflate the tourniquet to 250 mmHg after exanguinating the limb
- A 4 cm incision is made at the medial proximal aspect of the plantar fascia, at around 3 cm distal to the calcaneal insertion (**Figure 25.4**)

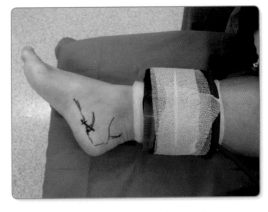

Figure 25.3 Patient positioning; supine position, external rotation of the limb, tourniquet at the ankle.

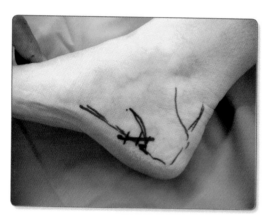

Figure 25.4 Skin incision at the medial aspect of the heel corresponding to the proximal insertion of the plantar fascia.

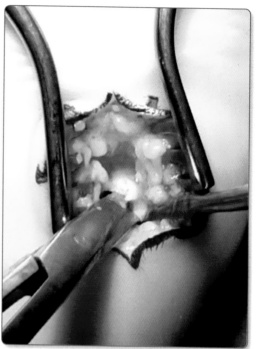

Figure 25.6 Cadaver specimen showing the insertion of the fascia on the plantar aspect of the calcaneum.

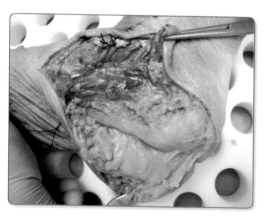

Figure 25.5 The plantar fascia is visualized.

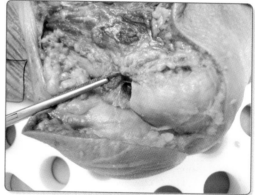

Figure 25.7 Cadaver specimen showing the site of the section of the fascia.

- Dissection is then continued until the medial band of the plantar fascia is visualized (**Figure 25.5**), and the inferior and superior margins are identified (**Figure 25.6**)
- Once the fascia is identified a transverse incision (**Figure 25.7**) is made through approximately the medial third of the fascia using either a no.15 blade or Mayo scissors, holding the hallux in maximal dorsiflexion (**Figure 25.8**)
- The plantar heel spur is palpated and is removed with a rasp. Removal of the spur is not always warranted. A large cadaveric study found that in about half cases, the bony spur

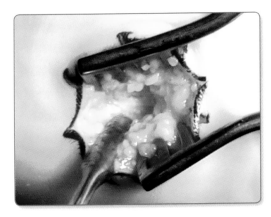

Figure 25.8 The plantar fascia is incised.

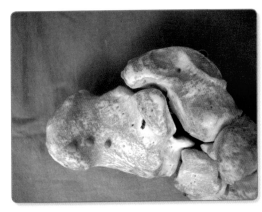

Figure 25.10 Site of bone perforations.

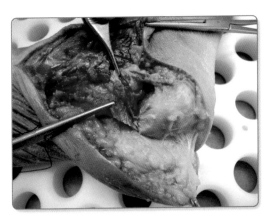

Figure 25.9 Detachment of adductor hallux tendon from the calcaneum in a cadaver specimen.

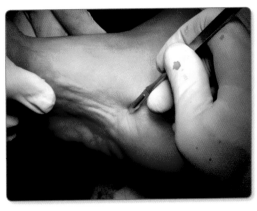

Figure 25.11 Percutaneous plantar fascia release.

was not in the same layer as the plantar fascia, suggesting that it did not have a causal role in the condition
- Optional procedures are:
  - Detachment of the adductor hallux tendon (**Figure 25.9**)
  - Infiltration of platelet-rich plasma
  - Bone perforation (usually three perforations of 3.5 mm diameter, in the plantar aspect of the posterior tuberosity) (**Figure 25.10**)
- No drainage is necessary
- Irrigation and hemostasis are applied

Surgical options

- A complete percutaneous procedure can be used (the same surgical steps but through a single small incision; use a no. 11 scalpel blade) (**Figure 25.11**)

Possible perioperative complications

- Bleeding

Closure

- Close the subcutaneous and skin layers in a standard fashion
- No drainage is necessary
- A simple dressing is applied

Postoperative management

Postoperative regimen

- Medication: NSAIDs, with thromboembolic prevention for 3 weeks

- Limb elevation for the first 48 hours
- Toe-touch weight bearing as the patient is able in the first week after the operation, progressing to full weight bearing after 2–4 weeks, according to tolerance
- Suture removal at approximately 2 weeks
- Outpatient visits on days 7 and 21 postoperatively

Early-phase postoperative complications

- Wound complications
- Infection

- Hematoma
- Complex regional pain syndrome
- Hypertrophic scar formation
- Osteomyelitis
- Calcaneal fracture
- Distruption of the medial calcaneal sensory branches of the tibial nerve
- Plantar fascia rupture
- Lateral column pain

Further reading

Celik D, Kuş G, Sırma SÖ. Joint mobilization and stretching exercise vs steroid injection in the treatment of plantar fasciitis: A randomized controlled study. Foot Ankle Int 2015 Sep 23 [Epub ahead of print].

Fallat LM, Cox JT, Chahal R, et al. A retrospective comparison of percutaneous plantar fasciotomy and open plantar fasciotomy with heel spur resection. J Foot Ankle Surg 2013; 52:288–290.

Gollwitzer H, Saxena A, DiDomenico LA, et al. Clinically relevant effectiveness of focused extracorporeal shock wave therapy in the treatment of chronic plantar fasciitis: a randomized, controlled multicenter study. J Bone Joint Surg Am 2015; 97:701–708.

MacInnes A, Roberts SC, Kimpton J, et al. Long-term outcome of open plantar fascia release. Foot Ankle Int 2015 Sep 8 [Epub ahead of print].

Surgical release of the superficial peroneal nerve

Indications

- Superficial peroneal nerve entrapment is a rarely encountered in clinical practice
- The indication for surgical release of this nerve is when a patient experiences symptoms resistant to pharmacologic interventions and the pain limits their ability to partake in sport and/or their usual activities of daily living

Preoperative assessment

Clinical assessment

- The patient describes pain on the dorsolateral aspect of the foot and ankle, classically with the exception of the first web space
- A painful 'trigger' point may be present in an apparently safe area, found 7–8 cm proximal to the tip of the lateral malleolus and anterior to the fibula. This is where the nerve pierces the deep fascia of the peroneal compartment and becomes subcutaneous
- Occasionally, if the nerve becomes entrapped in a surgical or traumatic scar, patients may experience painful triggering of pain at this specific site when it is knocked or occasionally when it is rubbed by tight-fitting foot wear
- If the lesion of the nerve is associated with axonal degeneration, either due to prolonged compression or trauma, a positive Tinel's sign may be found at the site of the site of entrapment
- A diagnostic injection using lidocaine administered at a specific 'trigger point' indicated by the patient's finger may help confirm this syndrome by resolving the symptoms for a number of hours

Imaging assessment

- Plain radiographs and ultrasonography investigations will likely be normal

- MRI may identify focal compression of nerve by a tight fascial band or by an area of fibrous scar tissue

Timing for surgery

- Surgery must only be performed in the absence of local inflammation and skin or soft tissue infections in the affected zone

Surgical preparation

Surgical equipment

- A basic surgical set with instruments for soft tissue dissection, such as curved Lahey forceps, and vascular loops

Patient positioning

- The patient may be set up in a supine position with a wedge under the ipsilateral hip to bring the foot into a neutral position. Alternatively, the patient may be set up in the lateral position, with the leg draped free to allow for intraoperative movement
- A tourniquet may be applied to the upper thigh. Alternatively, preoperative administration of local anesthetic with adrenaline (epinephrine) is accepted practice

Further preparation

- Preoperative antibiotic prophylaxis is not usually required

Surgical technique

- If a tourniquet is used, inflate it to 350 mmHg after exsanguinating the limb
- Make a vertical skin incision, centered at the site of maximal tenderness, approximately 7–8 cm above the tip of the lateral malleolus
- Isolate and protect the nerve with vascular loops before exploring proximally and distally for sites of compression (**Figure 26.1**)

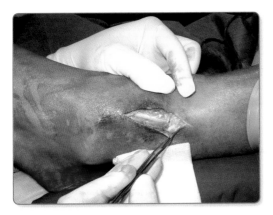

Figure 26.1 A tight fibrous band of scar tissue can be seen compressing the superficial peroneal nerve after it emerges from the deep compartment into the subcutaneous tissues.

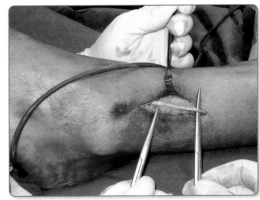

Figure 26.2 The fibrous band of scar tissue was surgically released, liberating the superficial peroneal nerve from further compression.

- After decompressing the nerve by releasing the overlying fascia or scar tissue (**Figure 26.2**), perform a neurolysis if necessary
- If recurrent, consider the use of biomaterials engineered to reduce the risk of new adhesions forming around the nerve as it heals

Possible perioperative complications

- Take great care to avoid causing an iatrogenic nerve injury, especially if the nerve lies in a bed of thick scar tissue

Closure

- No drainage is required
- Close the subcutaneous and skin layers in a standard fashion, avoiding any compression or traction on the nerve

- A simple dressing is applied
- Apply a posterior splint to prevent ankle movements and protect the wound

Postoperative management

- Nonsteroidal anti-inflammatory drugs and venous thromboembolism prevention (if high risk) are used up until full weight-bearing
- Elevate the foot in a cast for 2 weeks

Outpatient follow-up

- Day 14: Remove the cast, remove the sutures, mobilize the ankle, and reinitiate weight bearing

Further reading

Kernohan J, Levack B, Wilson JN. Entrapment of the superficial peroneal nerve: three case reports. J Bone Joint Surg 1985; 67:60–61.

Daghino W, Pasquali M, Faletti C. Superficial peroneal nerve entrapment in a young athlete: the diagnostic contribution of magnetic resonance imaging. J Foot Ankle Surg 1997; 36:170–172.

Yang LJ, Gala VC, McGillicuddy JE. Superficial peroneal nerve syndrome: an unusual nerve entrapment. Case report. J Neurosurg 2006; 104:820–823.